STUDY GUIDE TO ACC[...]

CONTEMPORARY MEDICAL-SURGICAL NURSING

Second Edition

Rick Daniels, RN, COL, PhD
Oregon Health and Science University Ashland, Oregon

Leslie Nicoll, PhD, MBA, RN, BC
Principal and Owner Maine Desk, LLC Portland, Maine

Prepared by
Dawna Martich, RN, MSN
Pittsburgh, Pennsylvania

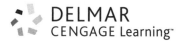

DELMAR
CENGAGE Learning™

Australia • Brazil • Japan • Korea • Mexico • Singapore • Spain • United Kingdom • United States

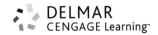
DELMAR
CENGAGE Learning™

Study Guide to Accompany Contemporary Medical-Surgical Nursing, Second Edition

Rick Daniels and Leslie Nicoll
Prepared by Dawna Martich

Vice President, Editorial: Dave Garza

Director of Learning Solutions: Matthew Kane

Executive Editor: Stephen Helba

Managing Editor: Marah Bellegarde

Senior Product Manager: Patricia Gaworecki

Editorial Assistant: Jennifer Wheaton

Vice President, Marketing: Jennifer Baker

Marketing Director: Wendy E. Mapstone

Senior Marketing Manager: Michele McTighe

Marketing Coordinator: Scott Chrysler

Production Director: Carolyn Miller

Production Manager: Andrew Crouth

Senior Content Project Manager: Kenneth McGrath

Content Project Manager: Allyson Bozeth

Senior Art Director: Jack Pendleton

Compositor: PreMediaGlobal

For product information and technology assistance, contact us at
Cengage Learning Customer & Sales Support, 1-800-354-9706

For permission to use material from this text or product,
submit all requests online at **cengage.com/permissions**.
Further permissions questions can be e-mailed to
permissionrequest@cengage.com

Library of Congress Control Number: 2010937557

ISBN-13: 978-1-4390-5863-3

ISBN-10: 1-4390-5863-6

Delmar
5 Maxwell Drive
Clifton Park, NY, 12065-2919
USA

Cengage Learning is a leading provider of customized learning solutions with office locations around the globe, including Singapore, the United Kingdom, Australia, Mexico, Brazil, and Japan. Locate your local office at: **international.cengage.com/region**

Cengage Learning products are represented in Canada by Nelson Education, Ltd.

To learn more about Delmar, visit **www.cengage.com/delmar** Purchase any of our products at your local college store or at our preferred online store **www.cengagebrain.com**

Printed in the United States of America
1 2 3 4 5 6 7 14 13 12 11 10

PREFACE

The second edition of the Study Guide to Accompany Contemporary Medical-Surgical Nursing by Rick Daniels and Leslie Nicoll is designed to facilitate student learning in clinical practice. Each of the 66 chapters covers issues relevant to the nursing profession: collaborative care, prioritization, and critical thinking to name a few. Questions are in a format similar to the NCLEX-RN® licensure examination including multiple choice, multiple response, fill-in-the-blank and sequencing.

By using this study guide in the clinical setting and classroom the student will work with the concepts important to medical-surgical nursing and understand how to apply those concepts to real-life nursing practice.

CONTENTS

UNIT 1 **Nursing and the Health Care System**   **1**

    Chapter 1 *The Health Care System and Contemporary Nursing*   3

    Chapter 2 *Clinical Decision Making and Evidence-Based Practice*   7

    Chapter 3 *Health Education and Promotion*   9

    Chapter 4 *Culturally Sensitive Care*   13

    Chapter 5 *Legal and Ethical Aspects of Health Care*   17

    Chapter 6 *Nursing of Adults Across the Lifespan*   21

    Chapter 7 *Palliative Care*   25

UNIT 2 **Supportive Patient Care**   **29**

    Chapter 8 *Health Assessment*   31

    Chapter 9 *Genetics, Genomics, and the Multiple Determinants of Health*   35

    Chapter 10 *Stress, Coping, and Adaptation*   39

    Chapter 11 *Inflammation and Infection Management*   43

    Chapter 12 *Fluid, Electrolyte, and Acid-Base Imbalances*   47

    Chapter 13 *Infusion Therapy*   51

    Chapter 14 *Complementary and Alternative Therapy*   55

    Chapter 15 *Cancer Management*   59

    Chapter 16 *Pain Management*   63

    Chapter 17 *Pharmacology: Nursing Management*   67

UNIT 3 **Settings for Nursing Care**   **71**

    Chapter 18 *Health Care Agencies*   73

    Chapter 19 *Critical Care*   75

UNIT 4 **Perioperative Patient Care**   **79**

    Chapter 20 *Preoperative Nursing Management*   81

    Chapter 21 *Intraoperative Nursing Management*   85

    Chapter 22 *Postoperative Nursing Management*   89

UNIT 5 **Alterations in Cardiovascular and Hematological Function**   **93**

Chapter 23 *Assessment of Cardiovascular and Hematological Function*   95
Chapter 24 *Coronary Artery Dysfunction: Nursing Management*   99
Chapter 25 *Heart Failure and Inflammatory Dysfunction: Nursing Management*   103
Chapter 26 *Arrhythmias: Nursing Management*   107
Chapter 27 *Vascular Dysfunction: Nursing Management*   111
Chapter 28 *Hypertension: Nursing Management*   115
Chapter 29 *Hematological Dysfunction: Nursing Management*   117

UNIT 6 **Alterations in Respiratory Function**   **121**

Chapter 30 *Assessment of Respiratory Function*   123
Chapter 31 *Upper Airway Dysfunction: Nursing Management*   127
Chapter 32 *Lower Airway Dysfunction: Nursing Management*   131
Chapter 33 *Obstructive Pulmonary Disease: Nursing Management*   135

UNIT 7 **Alterations in Neurological Function**   **139**

Chapter 34 *Assessment of Neurological Function*   141
Chapter 35 *Dysfunction of the Brain: Nursing Management*   145
Chapter 36 *Dysfunction of the Spinal Cord and Peripheral Nervous System: Nursing Management*   149
Chapter 37 *Degenerative Neurological Dysfunction: Nursing Management*   153

UNIT 8 **Alterations in Sensory Function**   **157**

Chapter 38 *Assessment of Sensory Function*   159
Chapter 39 *Visual Dysfunction: Nursing Management*   161
Chapter 40 *Auditory Dysfunction: Nursing Management*   165

UNIT 9 **Alterations in Immunological Function**   **169**

Chapter 41 *Assessment of Immunological Function*   171
Chapter 42 *Immunodeficiency and HIV Infection/AIDS: Nursing Management*   175
Chapter 43 *Allergic Dysfunction: Nursing Management*   179

UNIT 10 **Alterations in Integumentary Function**   **181**

Chapter 44 *Assessment of Integumentary Function*   183
Chapter 45 *Dermatological Dysfunction: Nursing Management*   185
Chapter 46 *Burns: Nursing Management*   189

UNIT 11 **Alterations in Gastrointestinal Function**   **193**

Chapter 47 *Assessment of Gastrointestinal Function*   195
Chapter 48 *Nutrition, Malnutrition, and Obesity: Nursing Management*   197
Chapter 49 *Upper Gastrointestinal Tract Dysfunction: Nursing Management*   199
Chapter 50 *Lower Gastrointestinal Tract Dysfunction: Nursing Management*   201
Chapter 51 *Hepatic, Biliary Tract, and Pancreatic Dysfunction: Nursing Management*   205

UNIT 12 **Alterations in Renal Function**   **207**

Chapter 52 *Assessment of Renal Function*   209
Chapter 53 *Urinary Dysfunction: Nursing Management*   211
Chapter 54 *Renal Dysfunction: Nursing Management*   215

UNIT 13 **Alterations in Endocrine Function**   **219**

Chapter 55 *Assessment of Endocrine Function*   221
Chapter 56 *Endocrine Dysfunction: Nursing Management*   223
Chapter 57 *Diabetes Mellitus: Nursing Management*   227

UNIT 14 **Alterations in Musculoskeletal Function**   **231**

Chapter 58 *Assessment of Musculoskeletal Function*   233
Chapter 59 *Musculoskeletal Dysfunction: Nursing Management*   235
Chapter 60 *Musculoskeletal Trauma: Nursing Management*   239

UNIT 15 **Alterations in Reproductive Function**   **243**

Chapter 61 *Assessment of Reproductive Function*   245
Chapter 62 *Female Reproductive Dysfunction: Nursing Management*   249
Chapter 63 *Breast Alterations: Nursing Management*   253
Chapter 64 *Male Reproductive Dysfunction: Nursing Management*   255

UNIT 16 **Special Considerations in Medical and Surgical Nursing** **257**

    Chapter 65 *Multisystem Failure* 259
    Chapter 66 *Mass Casualty Care* 261

Answer Key **263**

Nursing and the Health Care System

CHAPTER 1

The Health Care System and Contemporary Nursing

1. Before the 1800s, those who could not afford home care:

   a. Were assigned to sanitariums
   b. Were cared for in hospitals
   c. Were cared for in monasteries
   d. Were supported by the church

2. The use of engineering techniques to solve problems related to living organisms is referred to as _____.

3. During the 1960s, priorities of U.S. health care shifted to focus on:

   a. Efficient use of limited resources
   b. Health promotion
   c. Cost containment
   d. Illness prevention

4. The development of total quality management (TQM) and continuous quality improvement (CQI) was meant to:

   a. Assure society that cost containment would not compromise safety
   b. Serve as a system of external measures and balances
   c. Protect clients and their families during a health care crisis
   d. Result in extensive statistical databases for providing client care

5. The mission of the nurse and physician to relieve suffering and cure disease involved which of the following levels of care (select all that apply)?

   a. Sustain the client's life
   b. Attain client's enhanced health
   c. Regain the client's former level of health
   d. Maintain the client's former level of health

6. The Joint Commission (TJC) dimensions of quality performance identify _____ as the degree to which the risk of an intervention and risk in the environment are reduced for both client and health care provider.

7. The Health Insurance Portability and Accountability Act (HIPAA) focuses on:

   a. Providing universal health care to clients
   b. Protecting client confidentiality
   c. Decreasing the regulatory standards for medical documentation
   d. Improving administrative efficiency in documentation management

8. As senior hospital administrators, nuns were experts:

   a. In providing clinical care and managing resources
   b. At managing money and people
   c. Of health care and religion
   d. In none of the above

9. Historically, hospital administrators have come from various backgrounds. Please indicate the order in which members of each of the following groups have served:

   a. Physicians
   b. Nurses
   c. Nuns
   d. Businessmen

10. Nurses with advanced clinical knowledge coupled with business education were appointed as senior-level administrative officers beginning around the:

    a. 1940s
    b. 1950s
    c. 1970s
    d. 1980s

11. According to the American Nurses Association, the definition of professional nursing includes (select all that apply):

    a. A caring relationship
    b. Integration of research data
    c. Application of scientific knowledge
    d. Application of critical thinking
    e. Use of pay for performance criteria

12. The four domains of nursing are _____ _____, _____, _____, and _____.

13. Because of globalization and a health care environment charged with fear and ambiguity, nurse leaders must possess which of the following characteristics (select all that apply)?

    a. Competence in emotional intelligence
    b. Ability to optimize relationships
    c. Ability to resolve disputes under fire
    d. Competence to balance a unit budget

14. According to TJC, the "degree to which an intervention has been shown to accomplish the intended outcome" is referred to as:

    a. Efficacy
    b. Efficiency
    c. Appropriateness
    d. Effectiveness

15. Which of the following criteria are considered essential for a profession (select all that apply)?

    a. Possesses a specialized body of knowledge and skills
    b. Educates its practitioners in specialized graduate institutions
    c. Maintains a code of ethics that is enforced by colleagues
    d. Provides services that are vital to human and social welfare

16. The Doctor of Nursing Practice (DNP) program is intended to serve as a _____ degree for clinical nursing practice.

17. Modular nursing is based on:

    a. Work assignment by tasks to a group of clients
    b. Multiple caregivers of different educational levels
    c. Physical proximity of clients
    d. Case management and fiscal responsibility

18. Characteristics of the younger nurse include which of the following?

    a. Willing to sacrifice personal time when staff shortages arise
    b. Desire moderate amount of overtime work for increased salary
    c. Prefer to attend multiple-day professional conferences
    d. Unwilling to sacrifice family time to work overtime

19. Today's hospital environment is undergoing change. Which of the following changes are characteristic of contemporary work environments (select all that apply)?

    a. More natural light
    b. Interesting artwork
    c. Larger client rooms
    d. More noise because of technology

20. Collective bargaining agents, by law, can bargain over which of the following?

    a. Working conditions
    b. Benefits
    c. Salary
    d. All of the above

CHAPTER 2

Clinical Decision Making and Evidence-Based Practice

1. Sources of nursing knowledge include _____, _____ _____ _____, _____, and _____.

2. Research utilization promoted changes in practice based on:

   a. Studies of cause and effect
   b. Single research studies
   c. Quality improvement data
   d. Summary of evidence

3. Evidence-based practice has demonstrated that conclusions based on a body of research:

   a. Are more stable than results from a single study
   b. Require high-level analysis of data
   c. Should be viewed in the context of a clinical area
   d. Should be sufficiently narrow to be considered useful

4. Evidence-based practice operates on the basic premise that _____ is the most reliable source of knowledge on which to base clinical decisions.

5. According to the ACE Star Model of Knowledge Transformation, the steps necessary to move research from the bench to the bedside include which of the following (select all that apply and place in correct order)?

   a. Discovery
   b. Translation
   c. Integration
   d. Modeling
   e. Evidence summary
   f. Evaluation

6. Evidence summaries involve which of the following processes that help to yield more useful information for bedside practice (select all that apply)?

   a. Synthesis
   b. Application
   c. Intervention
   d. Meta-analysis

7. The first unique step in evidence-based practice is a(n) _____.

8. According to the Star Model, translation involves which of the following (select all that apply)?

    a. Considering the evidence summary
    b. Filling in information gaps
    c. Merging research knowledge with expertise
    d. Developing clinical practice guidelines

9. Examples of types of clinical practice guidelines may include (select all that apply):

    a. Clinical pathways
    b. Protocols
    c. Research expectations
    d. Algorithms

10. Single research studies never offer highly reliable answers to clinical questions.

    a. True
    b. False

11. Systematic reviews increase _____ and _____ of the cause-and-effect relationship between interventions and outcomes.

12. Typically, systematic review will require which of the following resources (select all that apply)?

    a. A 24-month schedule
    b. 6 to 12 investigators
    c. More than 3,000 articles
    d. $250,000

13. Two major sponsors of synthesis work are _____ and _____.

14. Which of the following entities most serves as an impetus for health care reform?

    a. National League of Nursing
    b. American Medical Association
    c. Institute of Medicine
    d. American Association of Colleges of Nursing

15. Production of evidence summaries is most likely accomplished by:

    a. The nurse at the bedside
    b. Clinical nurse specialists in practice
    c. Specialized, funded groups of scientists
    d. Health care provider researchers

Health Education and Promotion

1. The nurse would identify which of the following NANDA nursing diagnoses for a client who is in need of teaching?

   a. Ineffective coping
   b. Deficient knowledge
   c. Anxiety
   d. Fear

2. _____ , _____ is the communication of knowledge, values, behaviors, facts, and ideas relevant to the health status of the client.

3. To support the andragogy, the nurse should do which of the following when providing education to a client?

   a. Provide easy to prepare materials
   b. Focus on discussion as the primary teaching strategy
   c. Instruct on the day of discharge
   d. Set measurable goals

4. The nurse who instructs a client on the purpose of a medication is providing which of the following types of education?

   a. Formal
   b. Episodic
   c. Informal
   d. Ongoing

5. Discussion would likely be a desirable teaching strategy for the nurse who must teach:

   a. The newly diagnosed diabetic how to draw up insulin
   b. Childbirth classes
   c. The client with a joint replacement about anticoagulation
   d. A client how to turn, cough, and deep breathe

6. When giving a new mother a baby bath demonstration, the nurse can most effectively assess the mother's learning by:

   a. Asking her to give a return demonstration
   b. Having the mother talk about what to do
   c. Asking the mother to complete a short-answer quiz
   d. Having her practice on a doll

7. An effective means of teaching a young child about what to expect following surgery would be to employ:

    a. Demonstration
    b. Role playing
    c. Visual aids
    d. Computer-assisted instruction

8. Which of the following are characteristics of critical thinking (select all that apply)?

    a. Emotionally driven
    b. Organized
    c. Focused on positive health outcomes
    d. Isolated and competitive

9. The phases of the teaching–learning process include _____ , _____ , _____ , _____ , and _____ .

10. The nurse realizes that, to a large degree, the best teaching strategy for client education will depend on:

    a. The nurse's preference
    b. Assessment of the client's learning needs
    c. The client's diagnosis
    d. Time available for teaching

11. _____ , _____ is a significant factor in determining the type of information to be taught, the language to be used, and the location for teaching.

12. The nurse expects that the client is ready to learn when the client:

    a. Lies passively in bed during dressing changes
    b. Begins to ask questions about the healing process
    c. Moans constantly with discomfort
    d. Exhibits anxiety about how he or she will manage care at home

13. _____ , _____ is a client-centered and goal-directed form of counseling to assist a client make behavior change and achieve positive health outcomes.

14. A client tells the nurse that she learns best when she has an opportunity to try it out herself. The nurse realizes the client prefers which type of learning style?

    a. Visual
    b. Auditory
    c. Kinesthetic
    d. Affective

15. Which of the following are characteristics of health maintenance (select all that apply)?

    a. Perception
    b. Assessment
    c. Motivation
    d. Maintenance

16. _____ , _____ is the process of enabling people to increase control over their health and to improve their health by practicing behaviors that maintain or enhance well-being and avoiding unhealthy behaviors.

17. Which of the following global organizations takes the lead in developing education programs and policies to affect health promotion across the globe?

    a. World Health Organization
    b. American Medical Association
    c. American Red Cross
    d. Ministry of Health

18. Which of the following may be described by the nurse as being health-promoting behaviors (select all that apply)?

    a. Take a shuttle to work rather than driving
    b. Park farther out in the parking lot so one has to walk more
    c. Take the stairs rather than the elevator throughout the day
    d. Carpool rather than driving oneself to work

19. Which of the following are examples to support health promotion strategies?

    a. Recommend stress management courses for men
    b. Develop smoking restrictions after consulting with affected individuals
    c. Provide a teenage with a pamphlet about risky health behaviors
    d. Creating a women's club in a community

20. _____ , _____ , _____ is when client goals specified in the plan of care are reviewed and adjusted if necessary.

CHAPTER 4

Culturally Sensitive Care

1. Which of the following concepts help to define one's culture (select all that apply)?

   a. Employment
   b. Values
   c. Beliefs
   d. Attitudes

2. _____ refers to a group of persons whose members identify with each other through a common heritage.

3. Alienation, disorientation, or uncertainty that occurs during the process of adjusting to a new cultural group is considered _____ , _____ .

4. When assessing a client from the Native American cultural group, the nurse should include an assessment for which of the following disorders?

   a. Hypertension
   b. Cystic fibrosis
   c. Lactase deficiency
   d. Chronic liver disease

5. The nurse, caring for an African American client, realizes that one health belief within this culture would be which of the following?

   a. Illness can be punishment from God
   b. Illness is caused from pollution
   c. Illness is prevented by working
   d. Illness is caused by past events

6. Which of the following health values are often seen in an Asian American client?

   a. Deny themselves to care for elderly relatives
   b. Extended family is important
   c. Respect the past
   d. They are future oriented

7. The classification of a person based on shared traits such as body build, facial features, and inherited skin color is considered _____ .

8. The cultural group that is future oriented, competitive, and will not tolerate delays in health care is the _____ American.

9. For which of the following cultural groups might a client seek help from a curandero for an illness?

   a. Asian American
   b. African American
   c. Hispanic
   d. Native American

10. According to demographic data in the 20th century, which of the following ethnic groups has grown the most during the past 25 years in the United States?

    a. Hispanic (American)
    b. Asian (American)
    c. Pacific Islander
    d. Caucasian

11. According to data collected in the 2000 census, which ethnic group has been most concentrated in the Southern United States?

    a. Hispanic (American)
    b. Asian (American)
    c. African American
    d. American Indian

12. Which of the following should the nurse do when assessing a client who does not speak the same language as the nurse?

    a. Ask a family member to interpret
    b. Utilize a qualified interpreter
    c. Ask a hospital staff member who knows the language to interpret
    d. Ask another client who knows the language to interpret

13. In 2008, what percentage of homes in the United States reported speaking English "less than very well"?

    a. 10
    b. 20
    c. 25
    d. 30

14. Based on documentation of health disparities known to exist among different cultural and ethnic groups, which ethnic group suffers the highest mortality rates from cancer?

    a. Hispanic (American)
    b. Asian (American)
    c. Pacific Islander
    d. African American

15. A client immigrated to the United States 20 years ago. Which of the following would the nurse most likely assess for this client's health behaviors?

    a. Low or no smoking
    b. Limited alcohol intake
    c. Unhealthy diet
    d. No drug use

16. The nurse diagnosis that would be appropriate for a client who does not speak English would be:

    a. Altered verbal communication
    b. Impaired verbal communication
    c. Noncompliance
    d. Impaired social interaction

17. When delivering culturally competent care, the nurse should be _____, _____, and _____ .

18. When developing a plan of care for a client from a different culture, which of the following should be taken into consideration (select all that apply)?

    a. Preserve the cultural practices of the client
    b. Adapt the plan of care to address the client's cultural beliefs
    c. Instruct the client in White American health beliefs
    d. Repattern cultural practices that could be negative for the client

19. The cultural group that believes illnesses are treated with "hot" or "cold" foods would be:

    a. White American
    b. Native American
    c. Hispanic
    d. Asian American

20. Which of the following characterizes the middle-class American family structure?

    a. Less respect for authority
    b. Elders do not have a high position of respect
    c. Children have much value
    d. Focus is on self-responsibility and accountability

Legal and Ethical Aspects of Health Care

1. The nurse understands that one's worldview develops over a lifetime as a result of which of the following influences (select all that apply)?

   a. Socioeconomic status
   b. Religious background
   c. Family values
   d. Culture

2. _____ helps us to determine our beliefs about what is right and what is wrong based on our life experiences.

3. _____ refers to those ethical issues that impact a nurse's role in client care.

4. If an individual is at least 18 years of age and is capable of making reasoned choices, the nurse should assume that the person can make decisions regarding his/her own health care because the person has:

   a. Autonomy
   b. Demonstrated understanding
   c. Demonstrated ability
   d. Beneficence

5. The bioethical principle that implies that no harm should be done is likely to be of most use in which of the following situations?

   a. The client is a minor.
   b. The client is an elder.
   c. Further treatment may cause injury, pain, or harm.
   d. Denying treatment may result in death.

6. The ethical principle that suggests that nurses must contribute to the well-being of others is:

   a. Nonmaleficence
   b. Beneficence
   c. Justice
   d. Autonomy

7. The principle of clinical ethics that suggests that all people who seek health care should receive the best treatment available and that all people should be treated with dignity and respect is:

   a. Nonmaleficence
   b. Beneficence
   c. Justice
   d. Autonomy

8. The _____ code of ethics comprises nine statements intended to serve as a guide for practice.

9. The _____ is a code of ethics that describes what the client can expect from the health care enterprise and from health care providers.

10. When a nurse is aware of the right and moral action to take in a given client situation but is unable to perform that action because of external constraints:

    a. The nurse is liable to the client for damages.
    b. The institutional ethics board should be consulted.
    c. The nurse experiences frustrations inherent in managed care.
    d. The nurse experiences moral distress.

11. Which of the following scenarios is likely to lead to breach of client confidentiality (select all that apply)?

    a. Discussing care of a client in a hospital corridor
    b. Discussing care of a client in an institutional ethics committee
    c. Leaving a computer screen with client information visible to others
    d. Leaving printouts with client information lying where others may see it

12. According to the Health Insurance Portability and Accountability Act (HIPAA) of 1996, client information may be shared with which of the following individuals (select all that apply)?

    a. Health care providers involved in the client's care
    b. The news media
    c. Friends who call to inquire about the client's condition
    d. Family members designated by the client

13. A person who is younger than age 18 years but who is self-supporting and living independently is called a(n):

    a. Emancipated minor
    b. High school dropout
    c. Independent minor
    d. None of the above

14. Which of the following are considered forms of advance directives (select all that apply)?

    a. Living will
    b. Durable power of attorney for health care
    c. Verbal understanding between an individual and family
    d. Verbal understanding between an individual and the health care provider

15. The terms "palliative care" and "hospice" are interchangeable.

    a. True
    b. False

16. Barriers that hinder appropriate symptom management for clients near the end of life include fear of causing death of a client by administration of pain medication.

    a. True
    b. False

17. _____ is the term used to describe a situation in which the client's condition is such that aggressive therapy offers no medical benefit.

18. When a person has been assessed and considered dead by neurological criteria, the person is declared:

    a. Brain dead
    b. Legally dead
    c. To be in a persistent vegetative state
    d. None of the above

19. When a health care provider honors a valid request for a do not resuscitate (DNR) order, and the client consequently expires, the provider:

    a. Has participated in passive euthanasia
    b. Has performed a form of active euthanasia
    c. Condones assisted suicide
    d. Condones active euthanasia

20. Typically, an institutional review board might include which of the following individuals (select all that apply)?

    a. Health care providers
    b. Nurses
    c. Community members
    d. Clergy members

CHAPTER 6

Nursing of Adults Across the Lifespan

1. A client tells the nurse how "stressed" he is with life since changing jobs. The nurse realizes this client is within the adult stage of:

   a. Young adulthood
   b. The thirties
   c. Middle age
   d. Late adulthood

2. During an assessment, the nurse learns how the client associates health problems with different world events. This client is demonstrating which "time" of his development?

   a. Life
   b. Social
   c. Historic
   d. Psychological

3. The nurse is concerned about the upcoming influenza season. List the three components included when health issues are being tracked, recorded, and disseminated.

   a. _____
   b. _____
   c. _____

4. During morning report, the nurse notes that most clients are within his or her same age range. This observation is characteristic of:

   a. The nurse becoming older
   b. Less nurses available to work
   c. The nurse working on a pediatric unit
   d. The nurse making assumptions

5. The nurse is concerned that a client is at risk for suicide. Which of the following did the nurse most likely assess in this client (select all that apply)?

   a. History of alcohol abuse
   b. Recent death of a spouse
   c. Recent loss of full-time employment
   d. Family members moving near the client
   e. Joined a monthly reading club and weekly bridge club

6. When assessing an elderly client for compliance with prescribed medications, which of the following findings would indicate that the client is having financial difficulty?

   a. Forgetting to take the medication as prescribed
   b. Refusing to take the medication
   c. Cutting the medication in half and taking the medication on alternate days
   d. Taking the medication with pudding or Jell-O

7. Asthma is diagnosed most frequently in which of the following age groups (select all that apply)?

   a. Childhood
   b. Early adulthood
   c. Middle adulthood
   d. Late adulthood
   e. Old age

8. The nurse realizes that the leading causes of death for a 35-year-old client would be (select all that apply):

   a. Unintentional injury
   b. Suicide
   c. Congenital anomalies
   d. Respiratory disease
   e. Kidney disease

9. Which of the following can the nurse instruct an African American client to help control high blood pressure?

   a. Achieve a normal weight
   b. Reduce exercise
   c. Limit the intake of fruits and vegetables
   d. Maintain a fluid restriction

10. Before providing care to a client, the nurse sees that the client's blood glucose level is 112 mg/dL, waist circumference is 38 inches, and triglycerides are 220 mg/dL. Which of the following disease processes does this information suggest to the nurse?

    a. Chronic inflammation
    b. Arthritis
    c. Syndrome Y
    d. Metabolic syndrome

11. A client tells the nurse that she is scheduled for plastic surgery at a clinic that advertises procedures at half the rate of a plastic surgeon. Which of the following should be the nurse's response to this client?

    a. "I would like the name and telephone number of the clinic for myself."
    b. "Why do you want to have plastic surgery?"
    c. "The aging process is normal. Plastic surgery does not change that."
    d. "Make sure you know who is going to do the surgery and understand all the benefits and risks."

12. Bariatric surgery was conceptualized when which of the following surgeries were conducted?

    a. Coronary artery bypass
    b. Total hip replacement
    c. Gastric resection for peptic ulcer
    d. Carotid endarterectomy

13. _____ is a complex phenomenon comprising physical, functional, and psychosocial factors.

14. During the assessment of a client with coronary artery disease, the nurse wants to learn the client's modifiable risk factors. Which of the following would be considered such risk factors (select all that apply)?

    a. Blood pressure
    b. Mother having a heart attack at age 63 years
    c. Father dying of heart disease at age 41 years
    d. Smoking 10 cigarettes per day
    e. Cholesterol level 250 mg/dL

15. Which of the following have an impact on the daily activities of an elderly client?

    a. Cataracts
    b. Employment responsibilities
    c. Assisting with care of grandchildren
    d. Change in balance

16. A client comes into the clinic for an appointment seven years after having bariatric surgery. Which of the following findings would indicate this client's surgery was successful?

    a. Regained 50 percent of weight over the last five years
    b. Lost 60 percent of excess weight
    c. Only had three hospitalizations for abdominal wound infections
    d. Continues to need antianxiety medication

17. Which of the following characteristics would maximize the nurse's role when providing education?

    a. Serve as an advocate
    b. Build a trusting relationship
    c. Encourage to set unrealistic goals
    d. Limit teaching strategies used
    e. Knowledgeable of what motivates a person to learn

CHAPTER 7

Palliative Care

1. Hospice care is a coordinated program of service that delivers _____ rather than _____ .

2. The first modern hospice was developed in:

   a. Canada
   b. The United States
   c. England
   d. Italy

3. A checklist used to communicate therapeutic interventions the client does or does not want is:

   a. Required by law
   b. A power of attorney for health care
   c. A living will
   d. A legally binding document

4. A physiological state in which clients require a higher dose of drug to achieve the desired effect is:

   a. Physical dependence
   b. Tolerance
   c. Psychological dependence
   d. Addiction

5. The goal of palliative care is to (select all that apply):

   a. Relieve the client's suffering
   b. Control the client's symptoms
   c. Forego the client's curative therapy
   d. Support the client's functional capacity

6. In addition to support provided by the interdisciplinary hospice team, clients who opt to die at home must have a _____ .

7. The well-known psychiatrist who pioneered work on death and dying was:

   a. Florence Wald
   b. Cicely Saunders
   c. Robert McGill
   d. Elizabeth Kubler-Ross

8. Hospice care may be delivered in (select all that apply):

   a. The home
   b. An extended care setting
   c. A hospital
   d. An emergency department

9. The Medicare Hospice Benefit covers which of the following (select all that apply)?

    a. Hospital bed
    b. Around-the-clock care
    c. Medications
    d. Transportation

10. _____ refers to the practice in which a person other than the client provides medication to the client so that the client may commit suicide.

11. The states in which health care provider-assisted suicide has been legalized are (select all that apply):

    a. Oregon
    b. Utah
    c. Nevada
    d. Washington

12. Hospice volunteers perform which of the following activities for clients and families (select all that apply)?

    a. Shopping
    b. Respite care
    c. Bathing
    d. Assisting with activities of daily living (ADLs)

13. Dying clients may describe their chronic pain as:

    a. Intermittent
    b. Unrelenting
    c. Uncontrollable
    d. Rated 2 on a scale of 1 to 10

14. Which of the following are considered complementary and alternative medicine (select all that apply)?

    a. Acupuncture
    b. Music therapy
    c. Massage therapy
    d. Therapeutic touch

15. _____ refers to a practice in which someone other than the client directly administers medication that causes the death of the client.

16. Which of the following best describes the maximum dosage of opioid medication that may be administered for control of chronic pain?

    a. Morphine sulfate 10 mg per day
    b. Morphine sulfate 2 mg per hour as needed
    c. Morphine sulfate 1 mg per hour as needed
    d. Unlimited

17. Which of the following interventions would be beneficial to the dyspneic client?

    a. Placing the client in a prone position
    b. Placing the client in a supine position
    c. Keeping the room temperature cool
    d. Encouraging the client to sit in a chair

18. Which of the following bowel protocols would be most effective for the hospice client who receives high doses of opioids for pain control?

    a. Lactulose and enemas
    b. Bisacodyl and cascara
    c. Milk of magnesia
    d. Psyllium

19. During the last two weeks of a client's life, the nurse is likely to assess which of the following characteristics of the client?

    a. Increased urinary output
    b. Increased restlessness
    c. Improved communications
    d. Increased focus on religion

Supportive Patient Care

CHAPTER 8

Health Assessment

1. A client being seen for a peripheral vascular disorder in a health care provider's office would most likely need which of the following types of assessment?

   a. Comprehensive
   b. Emergency
   c. Ongoing
   d. Focused

2. The nurse is categorizing information collected during a focused interview. Which of the following is considered objective data?

   a. Pedal pulses present bilaterally
   b. Concerns about recent weight gain
   c. Increasing pain in the evening
   d. Heaviness in legs

3. Which of the following are considered secondary sources of data (select all that apply)?

   a. Literature review
   b. Client's family members
   c. Client's previous medical record
   d. Other health care providers
   e. Client-provided information

4. The nurse reviews and evaluates the progress of interventions toward intended goals. This describes which phase of the interview process?

   a. Orientation
   b. Working
   c. Intermittent
   d. Closure

5. During the assessment of a client, the nurse learns information about a client's immunizations, allergies, and medications. The category for this information is:

   a. Activities of daily living
   b. Management of health
   c. Sociocultural history
   d. Perception of health status

6. When assessing activities of daily living, the nurse would ask the client about which of the following (select all that apply)?

    a. Elimination patterns
    b. Family medical history
    c. Perception of self-identity
    d. Activity and exercise
    e. Sleep and rest

7. The _____ _____ incorporates the use of visual, auditory, tactile, and olfactory senses and the use of systematic assessment techniques.

8. Which of the following should the nurse palpate last?

    a. Triceps muscle
    b. Neck for cervical lymph nodes
    c. Ankles for edema
    d. Painful abdominal region

9. When auscultating for high-pitched sounds, the nurse should use the _____ of the stethoscope.

10. The nurse is preparing to conduct a physical assessment for a client. What four techniques will the nurse most likely use for this assessment (select all that apply)?

    a. Inspection
    b. Observation
    c. Percussion
    d. Palpation
    e. Auscultation
    f. Categorization

11. The nurse wants to assess the temperature of a client's edematous lower right leg. Which part of the hand would provide the best information for the nurse?

    a. Fingertips
    b. Dorsal aspect
    c. Ball
    d. Ulnar surface

12. Which of the following sounds are considered normal when using percussion over a client's abdomen?

    a. Tympany
    b. Flatness
    c. Dullness
    d. Resonance

13. A conscious learning process in which individuals become appreciative of and sensitive to the cultures of other people is considered:

    a. Cultural knowledge
    b. Cultural skill
    c. Cultural encounter
    d. Cultural awareness

14. Gender _____ is the masculine or feminine activities adopted by a person, which is often culturally and socially determined.

15. The selection and recombination of genes already existing in a gene pool is considered:

    a. Genetic screening
    b. Eugenics
    c. Genetic testing
    d. Genetic engineering

16. Which of the following can the nurse do to improve cultural competence (select all that apply)?

    a. Assume that all characteristics of a particular culture apply to those in the cultural group
    b. Develop an awareness of own existence
    c. Avoid cultural encounters
    d. Seek education in cultural competence
    e. Learn about other cultures

17. The nurse is reviewing ethical principles. List five principles of ethics seen in health care.

    a. _____
    b. _____
    c. _____
    d. _____
    e. _____

18. The nurse explains to a client how the information about his health status will be documented and shared. This is an example of:

    a. Health Insurance Portability and Accountability Act (HIPAA)
    b. Informed consent
    c. Advanced directive
    d. Advanced care planning

19. The nurse is documenting information gained from the assessment of a client. Which of the following would be considered subjective information?

    a. Blood pressure 136/84
    b. Facial grimacing when bending left knee
    c. Respirations 20 and regular
    d. Sharp, shooting pains in the right wrist

Genetics, Genomics, and the Multiple Determinants of Health

1. A client says, "My mother got diabetes when she turned 70. I guess when I turn 70 I will, too." Which of the following is the best response to make to this client?

   a. "That is right."
   b. "Not if you take measures, such as staying within your normal weight and exercising."
   c. "Only if your father has diabetes, too."
   d. "You are probably just a carrier."

2. A client who is three months pregnant is concerned that her baby will be born with Down syndrome because her sister's firstborn baby was born with the syndrome. Which of the following diagnostic tests could be prescribed for this client?

   a. Carrier screening
   b. Presymptomatic testing
   c. Prenatal diagnostic testing
   d. Conformational diagnosis

3. A female client is diagnosed with an X-linked recessive disease. Which of the following may occur if this client becomes pregnant?

   a. All children will have the X-linked disease.
   b. Only male children will have the X-linked disease.
   c. All children will be born normal.
   d. Only multiple births will have the disease.

4. The nurse is studying inheritance of traits. _____is the tool that is often used to illustrate homozygous and heterozygous traits.

5. A female client has an autosomal dominant inherited disorder. The nurse realizes this means:

   a. Every child born to this client will have the same disorder.
   b. Every child born to this client will have a 75 percent chance of inheriting the disorder.
   c. Every child born to this client will have a 50 percent chance of inheriting the disorder.
   d. Every child born to this client will be normal and not inherit the disorder.

6. According to the general principles of teratology, there are four types of abnormal cell development. List them.

    a. _____

    b. _____

    c. _____

    d. _____

7. A married couple is participating in genetic counseling. Which of the following are goals of this counseling (select all that apply)?

    a. Understand the genetic condition and how it is inherited

    b. Minimize the effects of the genetic deviation

    c. Adjust to family issues related to the genetic condition

    d. Provide information to aid with health care decisions

    e. Prevent the effects of the genetic deviation

8. The parents of a baby with a chromosomal abnormality are undergoing genetic counseling. How many generations of family history will this counseling include?

    a. 10

    b. 8

    c. 5

    d. 3

9. A female client has been identified as having "red flags" and is a candidate for genetic evaluation and testing. Which of the following are considered red flags for this client (select all that apply)?

    a. Marriage to an extended family member with one live birth

    b. First pregnancy at age 30 years

    c. Onset of menses at age 18 years

    d. Three miscarriages

    e. All male family members needing cardiac bypass surgery by age 35 years

10. A pregnant client is scheduled for a placental biopsy to identify any genetic defects in the unborn fetus. How many weeks gestation is this client most likely to be?

    a. 8 weeks

    b. 10 weeks

    c. 12 weeks

    d. 13 weeks

11. A client tells the nurse she is trying to become pregnant. Which of the following should the nurse assess in this client?

    a. Use of alcoholic beverages

    b. Number of siblings the client has

    c. Blood pressure

    d. Pedal pulses

12. A client comes into the clinic for a blood test to determine if she will develop a genetic disease that killed her father by age 45 years. The genetic blood test that has the highest degree of accuracy is the test for:

    a. Alzheimer's disease

    b. Multiple sclerosis

    c. Diabetes

    d. Huntington's disease

13. A client with asthma is concerned that any children he has will also develop the disorder. The nurse realizes genetic study is being done on this disorder; list the three major approaches.

    a. _____ _____

    b. _____ _____

    c. _____ _____

14. A client with sickle cell anemia asks about gene therapy for this disease. The nurse's response should be:

    a. "There are side effects, such as low platelets and red blood cells."
    b. "This was originally created to treat people with cancer."
    c. "It is in experimental stages right now, with positive results on mice."
    d. "You will have to take a medication to rid your body of excess iron."

15. A client who works in a chemical factory is concerned that unless he takes the employer's genetic test he will be fired. Which of the following responses would be appropriate to make to this client?

    a. "I would not take the test."
    b. "They want to increase your health insurance."
    c. "They want to see how much damage the chemicals are making to your body."
    d. "It might prove beneficial."

16. The nurse is a member of the hospital's ethics committee. List the four principles that support the ethical decision-making process.

    a. _____
    b. _____
    c. _____
    d. _____

17. The _____ _____ _____ _____
    (_____) prevents discrimination against anyone on the basis of their genetic information and prohibits health insurance companies and employers from using genetic characteristics as a basis for determining health services or hiring practices.

18. Which of the following is a benefit of pharmacogenomics?

    a. Create drugs based on specific diseases
    b. Base medication doses on a person's genetics
    c. Utilize viruses to introduce DNA codes into cells
    d. Eliminate the need for vaccinations

19. The oncology nurse is preparing a diagram of a client's family history in relation to cancer diagnoses. This nurse is constructing a:

    a. Histogram
    b. Pedigree
    c. Focused interview
    d. Genetic flow chart

CHAPTER 10

Stress, Coping, and Adaptation

1. While reviewing the most recent theories on disease and prevention, the nurse focuses on the biological module. From which theory did the biological model originate?

   a. Qi
   b. God's wrath on man
   c. Homeopathic
   d. Germ

2. While conducting a focused interview with a client, the nurse assesses stressors in the client's life. Which of the following are considered eustressors (select all that apply)?

   a. Buildup of carbon monoxide in the garage
   b. Accepting a new job with a company in a new city
   c. Spouse filing for divorce
   d. First child getting married
   e. Conflict with boss
   f. Taking a two-week vacation

3. The nurse is using the General Adaptation Syndrome to assess a client's level of stress. List the three stages of this syndrome.

   a. _____
   b. _____
   c. _____

4. The client says, "I just froze when I saw those two airplanes hitting the World Trade Center on September 11." The nurse realizes this client is describing the type of stress response often called "possum response" or _____.

5. A client tells the nurse how he reorganizes his day when he becomes overwhelmed with work and other responsibilities. The nurse realizes this client is using the following type of coping skills:

   a. Problem-focused
   b. Social response
   c. Emotion-focused
   d. Daily uplifts

6. A client practices alternative medicine approaches to help with the pain of arthritis. List five common complementary alternative medicine therapies.

   a. _____
   b. _____
   c. _____
   d. _____
   e. _____

7. During an assessment, the client states, "I have no big stressors in my life, just a bunch of small annoyances that don't amount to much." The nurse realizes this client:

   a. Is lucky
   b. Will be healthier than most
   c. Is stressed because of the cumulative effects of daily hassles
   d. Is in denial

8. A client says, "Whenever I feel stressed, I find a little time and write down what's bothering me in my journal." This client's activity is an example of:

   a. Maladaptive coping strategy
   b. Unconscious ego defense mechanism
   c. Repression
   d. Adaptive coping strategy

9. An elderly client tells the nurse, "I can't wait to go home." The nurse realizes this client is demonstrating which of the following characteristics:

   a. Denial
   b. Hope
   c. Spiritual well-being
   d. Adaptation

10. The nurse is assessing a client diagnosed with acute stress disorder. List the three symptoms of dissociation that this client may demonstrate.

    a. _____
    b. _____
    c. _____

11. A client asks about a pending thunderstorm and tells the nurse about all the hurricanes in Florida near her former home. The nurse realizes this client is demonstrating:

    a. Dissociation
    b. Posttraumatic stress disorder (PTSD)
    c. Anticipatory stress
    d. Burnout

12. A client diagnosed with PTSD is observed staring into space and not participating with any group activities. Which of the following characteristics of this disorder is this client demonstrating?

    a. Repressing the trauma
    b. Reliving the trauma
    c. Increased arousal
    d. Focusing on the cause

13. A client diagnosed with a chronic illness states, "I feel like there's no hope and wonder if living is worth it." This client is demonstrating:

    a. PTSD
    b. Dysthymia
    c. Anticipatory stress
    d. Dissociation

14. The nurse is providing care to a client demonstrating high anxiety. Which of the following interventions would be helpful for this client?

    a. Encourage sitting with other clients in the lounge area
    b. Encourage multiple family members to visit all at the same time
    c. Keep the client's room well lit
    d. Provide comfort measures and reduce noise levels

15. The daughter of an elderly client has a full-time job and travels to spend time with her family at least twice a week. Which of the following is this caregiver at risk for developing?

    a. Dissociation
    b. Psychiatric illness
    c. Caregiver stress
    d. PTSD

16. The nurse is reviewing information about stress management. Provide the name of the stress theory for each of the theorists listed.

    a. Roy = _____
    b. Neuman = _____
    c. Orem = _____

17. A client diagnosed with diabetes wants to reduce his blood sugar and increase his daily exercise. The nurse realizes this client would benefit from having:

    a. A personal trainer
    b. A dietary consult
    c. A social services consult
    d. A self-contract

18. The health care industry has undergone three revolutions over the past 30 years. List these three revolutions.

    a. _____
    b. _____
    c. _____

CHAPTER 11

Inflammation and Infection Management

1. The nurse is providing care to a client with an infection. List the two types of white blood cells responsible for conducting phagocytosis.

   a. _____
   b. _____

2. A client with an infection is demonstrating an activation of the clotting system. On assessment, the nurse will most likely observe:

   a. Increased circulation at the site of infection
   b. Reduced or no bleeding at the site of infection
   c. Phagocytosis at the site of infection
   d. Nothing

3. The nurse is assessing an infected leg wound. List the four signs of the inflammatory process.

   a. _____
   b. _____
   c. _____
   d. _____

4. A client has a history of chronic infections. Which of the following would be the body's attempt to heal this type of infection?

   a. Wall off the area with fibrous tissue
   b. Nothing
   c. Normal cell regeneration and return to full function
   d. Fill the area with a collagen fiber

5. A client is admitted with a urinary tract infection (UTI). The nurse realizes this health problem is an example of:

   a. A fungus causing a disease process
   b. A virus causing a disease process
   c. A bacteria causing a disease process
   d. A protozoa causing a disease process

6. A client is admitted with a disease caused by an inflammatory response. Which of the following is an example of this type of disease?

   a. Hepatitis
   b. Pneumonia
   c. UTI
   d. Arthritis

7. The nurse is planning care for a client with the nursing diagnosis: Risk for infection. Which of the following interventions would be appropriate for the nurse to include in the care of this client (select all that apply)?

   a. Pain management
   b. Use of standard infection control precautions
   c. Provide antibiotics
   d. Monitor white blood cell count
   e. Monitor for local and systemic signs of infection

8. The nurse is determining ways to reduce the introduction of infection into a client. List the five routes of transmitting microorganisms into a body.

   a. _____
   b. _____
   c. _____
   d. _____
   e. _____

9. The nurse is planning the care of a client with a wound that could splash or spray infected material. Which of the following protective items must the nurse wear when providing care to this client (select all that apply)?

   a. Sterile gloves
   b. Sterile gown
   c. Mask
   d. Eye protection
   e. Face shield

10. A client with an airborne transmission infection is being transported to radiology. Which of the following should be placed on the client before leaving the room?

    a. Sterile gown
    b. Mask
    c. Clean gloves
    d. Oxygen mask

11. A wound is healing with connective tissue that will not have the same capacity to carry out the normal tissue function. This type of healing is called:

    a. Repair
    b. Restoration
    c. Recovery
    d. Regeneration

12. A client is recovering from abdominal surgery. The nurse realizes this client's wound will heal by:

    a. Primary intention
    b. Secondary intention
    c. Tertiary intention
    d. Regeneration

13. A postsurgical client continues to smoke on discharge from the hospital. Which of the following will delay wound healing in this client?

    a. Lack of nutrients needed for healing
    b. Reduced inflammatory response
    c. Reduced blood flow to the area
    d. Stress on the scar tissue

14. A client had a knee replacement four days ago. In which phase of the healing process is this client now?

    a. Inflammatory
    b. Proliferative
    c. Remodeling
    d. Retraction

15. A client is demonstrating signs of delayed wound healing. List five reasons for delayed wound healing in a client.

    a. _____
    b. _____
    c. _____
    d. _____
    e. _____

16. The nurse is planning to assess a wound that is healing by secondary intention. How frequently should this wound be assessed?

    a. Daily
    b. With every dressing change
    c. Hourly
    d. Only when providing pain medication

17. The nurse is planning to use the Braden Pressure Scale to assess a client's risk for developing a pressure ulcer. List the six elements of this pressure scale.

    a. _____
    b. _____
    c. _____
    d. _____
    e. _____
    f. _____

18. The nurse is applying Opsite over a client's wound. Which of the following principles is the nurse implementing when managing this client's wound?

    a. Debridement
    b. Moist environment
    c. Prevent injury
    d. Nutritional support

CHAPTER 12

Fluid, Electrolyte, and Acid-Base Imbalances

1. The nurse is providing care to a client with extracellular fluid volume excess. List the three types of fluids within this compartment.

   a. _____
   b. _____
   c. _____

2. A client has a sodium and fluid imbalance. This client's body will attempt to regulate osmolality by:

   a. Increasing thirst
   b. Using osmosis and diffusion
   c. Increasing respiration
   d. Reducing urine output

3. A client is receiving an albumin infusion. This protein infusion will affect fluid balance by:

   a. Exerting oncotic pressure
   b. Exerting osmotic pressure
   c. Using diffusion
   d. Using filtration

4. A client with fluid volume excess has a low serum sodium level. This means the client:

   a. Needs a sodium chloride infusion
   b. Needs more oral fluids
   c. Has a diluted sodium level
   d. Needs a bicarbonate infusion

5. Physiologically, a client with fluid volume excess will have a stretching of the atria, causing the hormone _____ to be released.

6. The nurse is anticipating that a client with fluid volume excess will have an activation of the RAAS. RAAS means:

   a. R = _____
   b. A = _____
   c. A = _____
   d. S = _____

7. A client experiences a burn injury over 40 percent of his total body surface. The type of fluid imbalance this client is prone to developing is:

   a. Hyposmolar
   b. Excess
   c. Filtration malfunction
   d. Third spacing

8. A client has a blood urea nitrogen (BUN) to creatinine ratio of greater than 10:1. This means the client has:

   a. Third spacing
   b. Fluid volume deficit
   c. Fluid volume excess
   d. Nothing. This is normal.

9. Which of the following assessment findings suggests fluid volume excess?

   a. Drop in blood pressure with position change
   b. Thready pulse
   c. Sacral edema
   d. Positive pedal pulses bilaterally

10. A client with lower extremity edema has 8 mm of indentation. The nurse would document this finding as:

    a. + 1
    b. + 2
    c. + 3
    d. + 4

11. A client with heat stroke is diagnosed with hypernatremia. The cause for this client's disorder would be:

    a. Excessive water loss
    b. Excessive intake of sodium
    c. Excessive intake of chloride
    d. No particular reason

12. A client is diagnosed with heart failure. Which of the following could be a cause of hypokalemia in this client?

    a. Excessive sodium intake
    b. Stopped taking prescribed diuretics
    c. Excessive aldosterone release
    d. Wound drainage

13. A client is assessed with a normal potassium level. This means the client's potassium is between _____ and _____ mEq/L.

14. A client is prescribed the medication Spironolactone. Which of the following electrolytes will not be excreted with this medication?

    a. Sodium
    b. Potassium
    c. Chloride
    d. Calcium

15. The nurse has just performed two techniques to assess for hypocalcemia. List the two assessment techniques.

    a. _____
    b. _____

16. A client with chronic alcoholic intake and heavy antacid use is prone to developing which electrolyte imbalance?

    a. Hyperphosphatemia
    b. Hypophosphatemia
    c. Hypermagnesemia
    d. Hypomagnesemia

17. An elderly client recovering from surgery has a respiratory rate of 6 beats per minute. Which of the following is this client prone to develop?

    a. Respiratory alkalosis
    b. Respiratory acidosis
    c. Metabolic alkalosis
    d. Metabolic acidosis

18. Respiratory alkalosis can lead to which of the following electrolyte imbalances?

    a. Hypernatremia
    b. Hypokalemia
    c. Hyperphosphatemia
    d. Hypocalcemia

19. The nurse is beginning to determine the cause of a client's metabolic acidosis by using the _____.

20. The nurse is reviewing a client's arterial blood gases (ABGs). List the normal values for these gases.

    a. PO_2 = _____
    b. PCO_2 = _____
    c. HCO_3 = _____
    d. pH = _____
    e. O_2 Sat = _____

Infusion Therapy

1. Arteries and veins each have three basic layers. List these layers.

   a. _____
   b. _____
   c. _____

2. The nurse is preparing to administer packed red blood cells to a client. Which of the following intravenous solutions would be used during this transfusion?

   a. 0.9% normal saline
   b. Dextrose 5% and water
   c. Dextrose 5% and 0.45% normal saline
   d. Dextrose 5% and 0.9% normal saline

3. The nurse is determining where to place a venous access device on a client. Name the four veins the nurse can use on the client's hand or arm.

   a. _____
   b. _____
   c. _____
   d. _____

4. The nurse places an intravenous catheter in a client's cephalic vein. Which of the following is the client at risk of developing?

   a. Tissue damage
   b. Pain
   c. Deep vein thrombosis (DVT)
   d. Thumb numbness

5. The nurse is preparing equipment for a client's intravenous (IV) catheter and selects an add-on device. Examples of this device would be (select all that apply):

   a. Stopcock
   b. Filter
   c. Roller clamp
   d. Screw clamp
   e. Extension set
   f. Pinch clamp

6. Which of the following would the nurse assess in a client with an infiltrated intravenous line (select all that apply)?

    a. Redness
    b. Swelling
    c. Cool to the touch
    d. Redness
    e. Warmth
    f. Skin blanching

7. Which of the following can significantly decrease the risk of an IV-related infection?

    a. Transfuse D_5 water only
    b. Only use latex gloves when inserting the cannula
    c. Good hand washing
    d. Use clean gloves when inserting the IV cannula

8. A client experiences an extravasation. Which of the following should the nurse do (select all that apply)?

    a. Immediately remove the cannula
    b. Always apply a warm compress to the site
    c. Notify the health care provider
    d. Administer the identified antidote
    e. Compare the diameters of both arms

9. A nurse is using the formula method to calculate an amount of medication to provide a client. What does each of the following letters represent for this calculation?

    a. G = _____
    b. D = _____
    c. H = _____
    d. V = _____

10. To calculate a medication dose based on a client's weight in kilograms, the nurse could use the conversion of _____ pounds = 1 kilogram.

11. List the five rights of medication administration.

    a. Right _____
    b. Right _____
    c. Right _____
    d. Right _____
    e. Right _____

12. The home care nurse is providing IV medications for administration to a client in his or her home. Which of the following would be the nurse's responsibility for this medication therapy?

    a. Instructing client in self-administration techniques
    b. Mixing the medication
    c. Administering the medication
    d. Transporting the medication

13. List the four different modes of IV drug administration.

    a. _____
    b. _____
    c. _____
    d. _____

14. Clients with which of the following conditions would be considered candidates for central venous catheter placement (select all that apply)?

    a. Has an arteriovenous graft
    b. Prescribed eight weeks of IV antibiotic therapy at home
    c. Preoperative total knee replacement
    d. Need for replacement fluids short term
    e. Had axillary nodes removed for breast cancer

15. The nurse is preparing a client for peripheral parenteral nutrition. This client most likely:

    a. Has severe nutritional deficiencies
    b. Will resume regular eating in 1 week to 10 days
    c. Needs excessive nutritional supplements
    d. Only needs trace elements replaced

16. A client receiving a blood transfusion is demonstrating signs of a reaction. Which of the following would be early signs of a transfusion reaction (select all that apply)?

    a. Rash
    b. Thirst
    c. Chilling
    d. Fever
    e. Back pain
    f. Increased urine output

17. The nurse needs to start IV therapy in a 75-year-old female client. This client most likely will have _____ skin, _____ skin, and less _____ tissue.

18. A client is claiming a nurse was negligent when providing care. Place in order the following four conditions that must be present to prove this nurse's negligence.

    a. Breach occurs
    b. Damages and compensation
    c. Duty to act within a certain standard of care
    d. Breach causes harm

Complementary and Alternative Therapy

1. For which of the following disorders is complementary and alternative medicine (CAM) often used (select all that apply)?

   a. Joint pain
   b. Diabetes
   c. Asthma
   d. Back pain
   e. Neck pain

2. Which of the following are therapies within the field of traditional Chinese medicine (select all that apply)?

   a. Guided imagery
   b. Acupuncture
   c. Tai chi
   d. Biofeedback
   e. Qi gong

3. _____ is the practice of assisting in the health of clients through the application of natural remedies whereas _____ is the use of remedies without chemically active ingredients.

4. Complementary alternative therapy has roots in ancient peoples. List five cultures that have roots with this type of health care treatment.

   a. _____
   b. _____
   c. _____
   d. _____
   e. _____

5. The CAM therapy category that utilizes dietary supplements would be:

   a. Mind-body
   b. Biological
   c. Manipulative
   d. Energy

6. Which of the following are characteristics of a person who would use a CAM therapy (select all that apply)?

   a. Females more often than males
   b. High education level
   c. Males more often than females
   d. Low socioeconomic status
   e. High socioeconomic status

7. A client wants to begin a mind-body intervention. Which of the following would be this type of intervention?

   a. Chiropractic care
   b. Massage
   c. Guided imagery
   d. Reiki

8. Which of the following health conditions can be assisted with the use of biofeedback (select all that apply)?

   a. Headaches
   b. Scoliosis
   c. Hypertension
   d. Temporomandibular joint syndrome
   e. Arthritis

9. When using acupuncture, the needles assist in promoting the flow of _____
   or _____ along pathways known as _____.

10. The nurse should suggest that a client consult with an osteopath for which of the following health issues?

   a. Cancer
   b. Diabetes
   c. Appendicitis
   d. Carpal tunnel syndrome

11. A client asks the nurse what it "feels like" to have a chiropractic treatment. Which of the following should be the nurse's response to the client?

   a. "It hurts."
   b. "You will feel nothing."
   c. "You might have immediate relief of pain or mild muscle soreness afterwards."
   d. "It causes the same pain as having an injection."

12. A client tells the nurse that she didn't like the reiki session she had the other day because she felt exhausted and emotional afterward. The nurse realizes this client's reaction was due to:

   a. Being extremely ill prior to having the session
   b. The practitioner was not a Level III
   c. Reiki working on the physical, emotional, and spiritual levels
   d. The practitioner not being able to open the client's chakras

13. A client is planning to have deep tissue massage and manipulation to correct body posture. The nurse realizes this CAM treatment is considered:

   a. Acupressure
   b. Shiatsu
   c. Rolfing
   d. Reiki

14. Which of the following should be the nurse's instruction to a client who is planning on beginning herbal therapy?

   a. Study a good resource to select the best herbs to use
   b. Report herb use to the primary care provider
   c. Plan to take the herbs for several years
   d. Realize that herbal therapy rarely achieves effects

15. A client has been having reiki sessions. The nurse should instruct the client to:

    a. Ask to see the therapist's certificate of training
    b. Be sure the needles are sterile
    c. Not eat before a session
    d. Wear comfortable shoes

16. Which of the following are the physiological effects of humor (select all that apply)?

    a. Lowers cortisol levels
    b. Stimulates the release of catecholamines
    c. Exacerbates the immunosuppressive effects of stress
    d. Stimulates the release of endorphins
    e. Reduces hormone secretion from the pituitary gland

17. The CAM approach that uses "mind over matter" is considered _____.

18. Which of the following CAM approaches uses a group of people to hold their focused thoughts for healing on behalf of someone else?

    a. Intercessory prayer
    b. Guided imagery
    c. Reiki
    d. Meditation

19. Which of the following mind-body practices in CAM is used for a variety of health conditions and as part of a general health regimen to achieve physical fitness and relaxation?

    a. Shiatsu
    b. Rolfing
    c. Humor
    d. Yoga

CHAPTER 15

Cancer Management

1. The nurse is planning a client education class on cancer prevention. List the three factors known to contribute to the development of cancer.

   a. _____
   b. _____
   c. _____

2. Which of the following are characteristics of malignant cancer cells (select all that apply)?

   a. Uncontrolled cell division
   b. Specific morphology
   c. Poorly differentiated
   d. Migratory
   e. Euploid
   f. Cohesive

3. A client wants to learn how cancer develops. The nurse responds with the four stages of carcinogenesis. List the stages.

   a. _____
   b. _____
   c. _____
   d. _____

4. A client says he has never smoked. The nurse realizes this client has used:

   a. Primary cancer prevention
   b. Secondary cancer prevention
   c. Tertiary cancer prevention
   d. Restorative cancer prevention

5. The nurse is instructing a client about the warning signs of cancer using the acronym _____.

6. A client with cancer is receiving treatment to maximize his quality of life. This goal of cancer treatment would be:

   a. Cure
   b. Control the spread
   c. Palliation
   d. Preventive

7. The nurse is reviewing the most common treatments for cancer. List these treatments.

   a. _____
   b. _____
   c. _____

8. A client is going to receive implanted radiation for a large tumor before surgery. This radiation approach is called _____.

9. A client receiving radiation to his abdomen asks about side effects. Which of the following is an appropriate response for the nurse?

   a. There are no side effects.
   b. The side effects are worse than the cancer.
   c. Skin burns are the greatest side effect.
   d. You may experience bowel changes, nausea, and vomiting.

10. A client is prescribed chemotherapy after surgery to remove a cancerous tumor. The chemotherapy is used as:

    a. Brachytherapy
    b. Adjuvant therapy
    c. Neoadjuvant therapy
    d. Intracavity therapy

11. Chemotherapy can cause several side effects, including nausea and vomiting. Recently, research has found that the most distressing side effect to a client is _____.

12. An elderly client receiving chemotherapy is having difficulty initiating and maintaining sleep. Which of the following can the nurse do to assist this client?

    a. Ask the physician to prescribe a barbiturate
    b. Administer an antihistamine
    c. Encourage the client to engage in a light activity
    d. Administer an antidepressant

13. A client is prescribed a bone marrow transplant to treat cancer. List the three types of bone marrow transplant.

    a. _____
    b. _____
    c. _____

14. The nurse is caring for a client with cancer who is in a clinical trial for treatment. Which of the following should the nurse include in this client's plan of care (select all that apply)?

    a. Administer the treatment
    b. Provide emotional support
    c. Encourage the client to have an updated will
    d. Teach prevention of complications
    e. Encourage denial of the disease process

15. The nurse is planning care for a client who has fatigue caused by cancer treatment. Which of the following should be included as an intervention for this client?

    a. Encourage continuous increased activity
    b. Teach to minimize rest periods
    c. Assist with activities of daily living as needed
    d. Instruct on changing position from lying to standing

16. A client is neutropenic on the 12th day after starting chemotherapy. This means:

    a. The medication is working.
    b. Energy will return within days.
    c. Nothing
    d. The client is at a high risk for infection.

17. The nurse is concerned that a client being treated for cancer is developing a pleural effusion when which of the following is assessed?

    a. Dyspnea, restlessness, and chest pain
    b. Increased urine output
    c. Hematuria, petechia, and ecchymosis of the mucous membranes
    d. Acute change in mental status and respiratory distress

18. A client is prescribed Marinol to decrease nausea and vomiting from chemotherapy. The nurse realizes this medication is:

    a. A placebo
    b. An antianxiety medication
    c. A steroid
    d. Synthetic marijuana

19. Regarding body image, which of the following could the nurse suggest to a client with hair loss from chemotherapy?

    a. Nothing
    b. Many people look good without hair.
    c. It is permanent, so invest in wigs.
    d. Offer to call the Look Good Feel Better hair loss program for the client.

Pain Management

1. Pain is a(n)_____ interpretation of discomfort and is considered the_____ vital sign.

2. There are three theories to explain pain. List these theories.

   a. _____
   b. _____
   c. _____

3. A client complains of pain with venipuncture. Which of the following pain mechanisms does the entry of the needle into the vein represent?

   a. Transduction
   b. Transmission
   c. Modulation
   d. Perception

4. A client describes his leg pain as "throbbing." The nurse realizes the client is describing:

   a. Fast pain
   b. Slow pain
   c. Endogenous pain
   d. Pain threshold

5. A client with a large second-degree burn on his arm is not complaining of pain. Which of the following could be the reason for this client to not express pain?

   a. Client has a low pain tolerance.
   b. Client has a low pain threshold.
   c. The burn does not cause pain.
   d. Expression of pain is not accepted in his culture.

6. A client complaining of severe, right shoulder blade pain is diagnosed with gall bladder disease. This client's pain would be called:

   a. Pathological
   b. Neuralgia
   c. Nociceptive
   d. Referred

7. A client who experiences a transitory increase in pain that occurs in addition to persistent pain is experiencing:

   a. Breakthrough pain
   b. Acute pain
   c. Chronic intractable pain
   d. Neuropathic pain

8. Before prescribing treatment for a client's pain, the nurse reviews the five Cs of pain management. List these five Cs.

   a. _____
   b. _____
   c. _____
   d. _____
   e. _____

9. A client denies having pain, but the nurse has other assessment findings that indicate pain. Which of the following indicate the presence of pain (select all that apply)?

   a. Increased blood pressure
   b. Heart rate 68
   c. Restlessness
   d. Thirsty
   e. Anger

10. Which of the following would increase a client's risk for adverse reactions to NSAIDs (select all that apply)?

    a. 50 years of age
    b. History of gastric ulcer
    c. Currently prescribed warfarin
    d. History of cardiovascular disease
    e. History of osteoarthritis

11. The nurse is assessing a cognitively impaired client's level of pain with a scale that rates dimensions on a scale of 1 to 5. This pain assessment tool would be:

    a. Wong-Baker faces scale
    b. COMFORT Behavior scale
    c. Quality of Life scale
    d. PAINAID scale

12. A client is prescribed pain medication and asks for a dose yet does not appear to be in pain. What should the nurse do?

    a. Nothing. This client is addicted to pain medication.
    b. Offer a back rub instead
    c. Call the health care provider
    d. Provide the pain medication as prescribed

13. Which of the following is the best way to administer analgesics for a client with acute pain?

    a. Only when requested
    b. Around the clock
    c. Before meals
    d. At hour of sleep only

14. The nurse suspects a client has chronic pain because she is demonstrating the three Ss, which are_____, _____, and_____.

15. The nurse has decided the diagnosis of energy field disturbance is appropriate for a client. This diagnosis means:

    a. The client is addicted to pain medication.
    b. Nothing else fits the client's needs.
    c. The client had a CVA.
    d. There is disharmony of the mind and body/spirit.

16. A client with pain is prescribed an adjuvant medication. An example of this type of medication would be:

    a. Zoloft
    b. Aspirin
    c. Motrin
    d. Naprosyn

17. A client receiving an opioid analgesic is difficult to arouse and has constricted pupils. The nurse realizes this client is demonstrating:

    a. Pain relief
    b. Expected effects of the medication
    c. Overdose
    d. Drug toxicity

CHAPTER 17

Pharmacology: Nursing Management

1. The nurse realizes that oral medications undergo three phases before being used in a client's body and then eliminated. List these three phases.

   a. _____
   b. _____
   c. _____

2. During which phase is an oral drug disintegrated and dissolved for body absorption?

   a. Pharmaceutic
   b. Pharmacokinetic
   c. Pharmacodynamic
   d. Distribution

3. Once used by the body, oral medications must be detoxified to be cleared from the body. This process of pharmacokinetics is:

   a. Absorption
   b. Distribution
   c. Biotransformation
   d. Excretion

4. _____ describes the biological and physiological effects a drug has on the body.

5. The nurse is preparing to administer a medication to a client. Place in order the following "rights" of medication administration the nurse should follow.

   a. Right drug
   b. Right time
   c. Right dose
   d. Right client
   e. Right documentation
   f. Right route

6. Before giving a drug to a client, how many checks should the nurse do to ensure safety?

   a. One
   b. Two
   c. Three
   d. Four

7. During the assessment of an elderly client, the nurse learns the client takes Lasix 20 mg by mouth (PO) and Furosemide 40 mg PO every morning. This finding suggests:

    a. History of urinary retention
    b. Polypharmacy
    c. Well-functioning cardiovascular status
    d. Nothing

8. A client is prescribed a medication that the nurse has never administered. Which of the following should the nurse do?

    a. Ask another nurse about the drug
    b. Give the client the drug
    c. Refuse to give the drug
    d. Research the drug before giving it to the client

9. The nurse learns a client has an allergy to penicillin. Which of the following classes of anti-infectives should not be prescribed for this client?

    a. Cephalosporins
    b. Macrolides
    c. Tetracyclines
    d. Fluoroquinolones

10. A client is ordered peak-and-trough venous blood levels drawn. Which of the following anti-infectives is the client most likely receiving?

    a. Cephalosporin
    b. Aminoglycoside
    c. Macrolide
    d. Tetracycline

11. An elderly client on 0.125 mg digoxin complains of vision changes and diarrhea. Which of the following should be done for this client?

    a. Nothing. This is normal.
    b. Provide an antidiarrheal medication
    c. Schedule an eye examination
    d. Draw a digoxin level checking for toxicity

12. A client is prescribed a beta-blocker. Which of the following should the nurse include when instructing this client (select all that apply)?

    a. If pain continues after three doses, call 911.
    b. Change positions slowly.
    c. Stop smoking.
    d. Take an extra dose before exercising.
    e. Expect a weight gain when taking this medication.
    f. Stop taking this medication if dizziness develops.

13. A client has been taking aldactone and an angiotensin-converting enzyme (ACE) inhibitor. Which of the following is this client at risk of developing?

    a. Hyponatremia
    b. Hypercalcemia
    c. Hyperkalemia
    d. Nothing

14. A client is receiving a heparin infusion for a deep vein thrombosis (DVT). Which of the following blood tests will be performed to determine the effectiveness of this medication?

    a. Activated partial thromboplastin time (APTT)
    b. APTT and prothrombin time (PT)
    c. APTT and international normalized ratio (INR)
    d. APTT, PT, and INR

15. Which of the following medications would be indicated for a client with chronic asthma?

    a. Atrovent
    b. Isuprel
    c. Alupent
    d. Serevent

16. A client with seizures is started on Dilantin. Which of the following should the nurse include when instructing this client (select all that apply)?

    a. Urine may turn pink, red, or brown
    b. Use alcohol in moderation
    c. Substitute a generic brand if the trade brand is unavailable
    d. Brush teeth with a soft toothbrush
    e. Double the dose of oral birth control pills

17. A client is diagnosed with gastroesophageal reflux disease (GERD). Which of the following medications are effective for this health condition (select all that apply)?

    a. Cimetidine
    b. Aspirin
    c. Axid
    d. Zantac
    e. Pepcid

18. Which of the following types of insulin can be administered intravenously?

    a. Regular
    b. NPH
    c. Human
    d. Beef

19. A client with type 2 diabetes mellitus is prescribed a medication that will slow the effectiveness of the enzyme needed to digest carbohydrates. Which of the following medications will do this?

    a. Orinase
    b. Precose
    c. Dymelor
    d. Glynase

Settings for Nursing Care

CHAPTER 18

Health Care Agencies

1. To achieve the goal of providing health care to all citizens, the core values of _____, _____, and _____ must be addressed.

2. Which of the following are publicly funded health insurance plans (select all that apply)?

   a. Medicare
   b. Health Maintenance Organization (HMO)
   c. Preferred Provider Organization (PPO)
   d. Medicaid
   e. Department of Veterans Affairs

3. List the five components that impact access to health care.

   a. _____
   b. _____
   c. _____
   d. _____
   e. _____

4. A hospital is using Donabedian's framework to evaluate the quality of care. List the three variables in this framework.

   a. _____
   b. _____
   c. _____

5. Outcome variables are the result of care delivered and can be categorized as being _____, _____, and _____.

6. The purpose of a health care agency that focuses on prevention is to:

   a. Provide specialized care
   b. Provide basic routine care
   c. Provide inclient treatment only
   d. Provide education

7. Which of the following would be considered a primary care agency?

   a. Urgent care center
   b. Rehabilitation hospital
   c. Psychiatric hospital
   d. Assisted living facility

8. Which of the following would be considered secondary health care agencies (select all that apply)?

   a. Trauma center
   b. Ambulatory clinic
   c. Pediatric hospital
   d. Community hospital that performs surgeries
   e. Organ transplant hospital

9. Which of the following types of health care agencies is an important site for educating and training future health care professionals?

    a. Preventive care
    b. Primary care
    c. Secondary care
    d. Tertiary care

10. _____ _____ facilities provide health, social, and recreational services to adults who require supervision and care while their family members are at work.

11. Of the following, choose those that are considered restorative health care agencies (select all that apply).

    a. Home care
    b. Burn unit
    c. Skilled nursing facility
    d. Inpatient surgical unit
    e. Rehabilitation hospital

12. A client with a chronic debilitating illness would best be served by which of the following types of health care agencies?

    a. Tertiary care
    b. Quaternary care
    c. Restorative care
    d. Continuing care

13. The Center for Medicare/Medicaid Services monitors regulatory compliance of nursing homes by using two data sets. List these two data sets.

    a. _____
    b. _____

14. An ideal health care system provides seamless care through comprehensive disease management. One example of this new model of care delivery would be:

    a. Case management
    b. Integrated care delivery
    c. Primary nursing
    d. Holistic care delivery

15. The Synergy Model of patient care makes the assumption that client _____ and nurse _____ match.

16. How many nursing competencies are defined within the Synergy Model of patient care?

    a. 10
    b. 8
    c. 6
    d. 4

17. What does each of the letters represent within the SBAR communication technique?

    S = _____
    B = _____
    A = _____
    R = _____

18. The concept of safe passage within the Synergy Model of patient care means:

    a. Safe transportation between departments in a hospital
    b. Safely return home after discharge from a hospital
    c. Client safety and excellent practice
    d. Nothing in today's health care agencies

CHAPTER 19

Critical Care

1. List the two types of critical care units.

   a. _____
   b. _____

2. Which of the following abbreviations can a nurse use after his or her name after passing the American Association of Critical Nursing critical care examination?

   a. RN, CC
   b. CCRN
   c. CCNS
   d. RN, C

3. Which of the following assessment findings would identify a client for admission to a critical care unit (select all that apply)?

   a. Electrocardiogram (ECG) findings of an acute myocardial infarction
   b. Serum potassium level 3.2 mg/dL
   c. Blood pressure 168/88 mm Hg
   d. Cervical spine fracture
   e. Body temperature 97.9° F (36.6° C)
   f. Needing mechanical ventilation

4. Sleep deprivation is common for clients in critical care units. Which of the following can be done to help reduce this problem?

   a. Restrict visitors
   b. Play music
   c. Minimize any unnecessary lighting
   d. Perform passive range of motion on lower extremities every two hours

5. List the five principal needs of a family with a client in the critical care area.

   a. _____
   b. _____
   c. _____
   d. _____
   e. _____

6. Which of the following would help the families of critical care clients (select all that apply)?

   a. Send them home to sleep
   b. Permit visitation when possible
   c. Restrict visitation to 15 minutes every four hours
   d. Contact social services or pastoral care if requested and needed
   e. Explain what is happening with the client
   f. Tell them the doctor will talk with them

7. A client needs hemodynamic monitoring. Which of the following are the most common complications of this monitoring (select all that apply)?

   a. Infection
   b. Pulmonary embolism
   c. Deep vein thrombosis
   d. Paralytic ileus
   e. Bleeding

8. Which of the following is a device to measure cardiac output and central venous pressure?

   a. Intra-aortic balloon
   b. Femoral arterial line
   c. Pulmonary artery catheter
   d. Percutaneously inserted central catheter (PICC) line

9. The nurse notes an overdamping of a waveform on a client with hemodynamic monitoring. To correct this problem, list what the nurse should check for.

   a. _____
   b. _____
   c. _____
   d. _____

10. During the placement of a Swan Ganz catheter through the right ventricle, which of the following can occur?

    a. Increase in blood pressure
    b. Persistent coughing
    c. No bowel sounds
    d. Ventricular arrhythmias

11. A client experiencing hypotension needs a mean arterial pressure (MAP) of at least _____ mm Hg to perfuse organs.

12. Which of the following are indications that a client is not a candidate for an intra-aortic balloon pump (select all that apply)?

    a. Severe peripheral vascular disease
    b. Dissecting abdominal aortic aneurysm
    c. Precoronary artery bypass surgery
    d. No femoral pulses
    e. Cardiogenic shock

13. Active monitoring of the color, temperature, and pulse of the appropriate extremity on a client with an intra-aortic balloon will:

    a. Ensure sufficient cerebral tissue perfusion
    b. Prevent the catheter from kinking
    c. Help prevent immobility complications
    d. Prevent dislodgement of the balloon

14. A client with a(n) _____ _____ _____ may be discharged to home after caregivers receive education regarding equipment, alarms, and emergency situations.

15. On analysis of a client with an intracranial monitoring device's waveform, the nurse calls for help. Which of the waveforms did this nurse likely see?

    a. A waves only
    b. A waves or B waves
    c. B waves only
    d. C waves

16. To facilitate venous drainage for a client with an intracranial pressure device, the nurse should maintain the client's head of the bed at which of the following degrees of elevation?

    a. 60
    b. 45
    c. 10
    d. 0

17. When placing an endotracheal tube through the mouth, the client's head should be placed in the _____ position.

18. A client who requires long-term ventilator support would benefit from which type of oxygen delivery system?

    a. Tracheostomy
    b. Endotracheal tube
    c. Nasotracheal tube
    d. Transtracheal approach

19. A client who is spontaneously breathing after anesthesia but has a history of sleep apnea would benefit from which type of ventilator support?

    a. Positive end expiratory pressure (PEEP)
    b. Pressure controlled ventilation
    c. Continuous positive airway pressure (CPAP)
    d. Mandatory minute ventilation

20. Which of the following should be included when providing care to a client who is mechanically ventilated (select all that apply)?

    a. Keep ventilator alarms on
    b. Suction for 30 to 45 seconds
    c. Continuous pulse oximetry monitoring
    d. Ambu bag and mask at the bedside
    e. Position bed in Trendelenburg
    f. Monitor endotracheal tube cuff pressure at least once per shift

Perioperative Patient Care

CHAPTER 20

Preoperative Nursing Management

1. List the two developments that have aided the planning for surgery, hastened a client's recovery, and satisfied insurers.

   a. _____

   b. _____

2. _____-_____ _____ describes a procedure that a client receives in one day and in which he or she is discharged within 23 hours of admission.

3. Which of the following indicates that a hospital has the most excellent nursing care?

   a. Rural facility
   b. City or county hospital
   c. University affiliation
   d. Magnet status

4. Of the following, choose those that describe elective surgery (select all that apply):

   a. Emergency in nature
   b. No urgency
   c. Needed to recover from an accident
   d. Adequate time for teaching
   e. Time to plan
   f. Lifesaving surgery

5. A client is scheduled for surgery in one week. The client should be instructed to:

   a. Eat nutritious meals
   b. Cut calories to lose some weight
   c. Increase exercise
   d. Avoid sleeping for more than five hours each night

6. A nurse who witnesses a client sign a surgical consent form is witnessing that:

   a. The client understands the surgery to be performed.
   b. The health care provider explained the procedure to the client.
   c. The client knows how to write.
   d. The client is capable of giving consent without coercion.

7. The nurse who managed the care of a client during the direct surgical experience is called the _____ nurse.

8. The nurse observes a preoperative surgical client's family member writing down information on a pad of paper. Which of the following should the nurse do about this observation?

   a. Ask the family member to stop writing
   b. Tell the family, "It is my word against yours."
   c. Nothing. This is fine.
   d. Refuse to care for the client

9. An elderly client in the surgical holding area is waiting to go to surgery. Which of the following can the nurse do to help this client?

   a. Rush through the preoperative activities
   b. Give the client a glass of water
   c. Slow the pace of activities
   d. Speak loudly because elderly clients always have hearing loss

10. Which of the following clients are at risk for hypothermia during a surgical procedure (select all that apply)?

   a. 90-year-old client having a colon resection
   b. 35-year-old client having carpal tunnel surgery
   c. 41-year-old client having arthroscopic knee surgery
   d. 60-year-old client prescribed warfarin for atrial fibrillation
   e. 75-year-old client having total hip replacement surgery

11. A client is scheduled for a right total knee replacement. Which of the following would ensure proper surgical site identification?

   a. Apply an ACE bandage over the left knee
   b. Apply an ACE bandage over the right knee
   c. Draw a smiley face over the right knee
   d. Mark YES over the right knee

12. The nurse is preparing preoperative medications for a client. List the four categories of these medications.

   a. _____
   b. _____
   c. _____
   d. _____

13. Which of the following client characteristics present possible challenges for care in the preoperative period (select all that apply)?

   a. No drug allergies
   b. Previous orthopedic surgeries
   c. Alcohol intake of more than three drinks per day
   d. Weight 25 percent over normal
   e. Family member monitoring activities
   f. Recent history of smoking

14. The health care providers discover that a client has a blood vessel leaking blood into the abdominal cavity. The type of surgery this client needs is characterized as being _____.

15. In the case of emergency surgery, which of the following statuses has the highest priority?

   a. Psychosocial
   b. Physical
   c. Spiritual
   d. Socioeconomic

16. The nurse suspects a client may have an allergy to latex when which of the following is assessed (select all that apply)?

    a. Multiple hospitalizations
    b. Allergic to house dust
    c. Allergic to specific foods
    d. History of eczema
    e. History of lactose intolerance

17. The client who self-donates blood prior to an elective surgical procedure is participating in _____ donation.

CHAPTER 21

Intraoperative Nursing Management

1. Which of the following surgical team members works directly with the surgeon, providing instruments and other items during the procedure?

   a. Circulating nurse
   b. Scrub nurse
   c. Registered nurse first assistant
   d. Surgical technologist

2. A client with spinal stenosis needs surgery. In which of the surgical specialties could this procedure be categorized (select all that apply)?

   a. General
   b. Neurological
   c. Gynecological
   d. Thoracic
   e. Orthopedic

3. A client is scheduled for a carotid endarterectomy. This is considered a(n) _____-risk surgical procedure.

4. Which of the following is of particular concern when providing care to a pediatric surgical client?

   a. Pain control
   b. Length of hospital stay
   c. Amount of toys the child can have
   d. Performing surgical wound dressing changes at home

5. A client with Parkinson's disease is scheduled for a total hip replacement. Which of the following interventions would be helpful for this client (select all that apply)?

   a. Continuous cardiac monitoring
   b. Thrombosis prophylaxis
   c. Monitor blood glucose levels every four hours
   d. Ensure a weighted feeding tube is placed for medication administration
   e. Assess oxygenation level
   f. Medicate for pain around the clock

6. Most surgical suites are divided into three areas based on the activities within each area. List these areas.

   a. _____
   b. _____
   c. _____

7. A surgical instrument will be used to penetrate soft tissue. According to the Spaulding sterilization system, this instrument is classified as being:

   a. Critical
   b. Semicritical
   c. Noncritical
   d. None of the above

8. _____ is a process that destroys all microorganisms, whereas _____ destructs or inhibits most pathogens on inanimate objects.

9. A nurse is putting on a sterilized surgical gown to assist with a surgical procedure. Which areas of the gown are considered sterile (select all that apply)?

   a. Front of chest to the level of the sterile field
   b. Entire neck area
   c. Both sleeves from the cuff to slightly above the elbow
   d. Shoulders and underarms
   e. Back of the gown
   f. Entire gown

10. A scrub nurse notices a tear on the right ring finger of the sterile glove. What should the nurse do?

    a. Avoid touching anything with the right hand
    b. Ask the circulating nurse to remove the glove
    c. Take off the gloves and place them on the sterile field
    d. Remove gloves, wash hands, and apply sterile gloves

11. The purposes of electrosurgery are to cut, _____, or _____ tissue.

12. Which of the following will depress consciousness while permitting the client to respond purposefully to verbal commands?

    a. General anesthesia
    b. Local anesthesia
    c. Conscious sedation
    d. Deep conscious sedation

13. List the five types of anesthesia.

    a. _____
    b. _____
    c. _____
    d. _____
    e. _____

14. Which of the following describes when it is appropriate to perform surgical counts?

    a. Count sponges at the end of the procedure only
    b. Count sponges before the procedure to establish a baseline
    c. It is not necessary to count sharps
    d. Instruments are counted only when changing the scrub nurse

15. Which of the following indicate that a surgical client is at risk for developing malignant hyperthermia (select all that apply)?

    a. Low sodium level
    b. Evidence of metabolic acidosis
    c. Elevated potassium level
    d. Bradycardia
    e. Presence of masseter spasm

16. The circulating nurse should initiate a _____ _____ to verify the correct client, procedure, site, side, surgeon, position, and equipment.

17. Which regulatory body publishes National Patient Safety Goals that have direct implications for surgical care?

    a. The Joint Commission (TJC)
    b. CARF
    c. American Association of Critical Nursing
    d. CMS

18. Which of the following are considered risks of anesthesia (select all that apply)?

    a. Nausea and vomiting
    b. Sore throat
    c. Urinary tract infection
    d. Heart attack
    e. Pneumonia

CHAPTER 22

Postoperative Nursing Management

1. Which of the following are reasons postsurgical care has improved since World War II (select all that apply)?

   a. Improved technology
   b. Specialized training for nurses
   c. Returning clients to the general unit after surgery
   d. Individualized client care resulting from nursing staff levels in the postanesthesia critical unit (PACU)
   e. More trained surgeons

2. A client is discharged from surgery and is admitted directly into the surgical intensive care unit (ICU). Which of the following would ensure that this client receives the highest quality of care?

   a. Assign a PACU nurse to provide care in the surgical ICU
   b. Make sure the client's airway is patent
   c. Cross-train all surgical ICU nurses in recovery from surgery and anesthesia
   d. Have the surgical ICU nurse review the newest National Patient Safety goals

3. A client had a surgical procedure that lasted 45 minutes. Into which of the following care areas is this client most likely to be admitted to recover from the surgery?

   a. Critical care unit
   b. Surgical ICU
   c. General surgery ward
   d. PACU with plan to discharge to home

4. In which of the following ways has the enactment of Health Insurance Portability and Accountability Act (HIPAA) legislation impacted the PACU?

   a. Clipboards must be kept visible at the foot of the bed.
   b. Not all clients can have family with them in the PACU.
   c. Report must occur at the bedside.
   d. Two nurses must check the client's postsurgical orders.

5. A nurse is admitting a client into the PACU. Of the following, choose the areas that will receive the most assessment attention regardless of the surgical procedure (select all that apply)?

   a. Respiratory stability
   b. Bowel sounds
   c. Ability to swallow
   d. Surgical site
   e. Nausea and vomiting
   f. Cardiac stability

6. A nurse is planning to use a special type of blanket that has pockets filled with warm, circulating air to help warm a client after surgery. This blanket is called a(n) _____ _____.

7. Which of the following can the nurse do when planning care for an elderly client recovering from surgery?

   a. Encourage the completion of care activities in a set amount of time
   b. Refer to the client by his or her first name
   c. Turn on the overhead lights when entering the room
   d. Permit the client time to respond to questions because of a hearing deficit

8. List the three types of drains placed into a surgical wound.

   a. _____
   b. _____
   c. _____

9. The _____ _____ is a system that is used to assess a client's readiness to be discharged from the PACU.

10. Which of the following should a client do postoperatively to prevent atelectasis?

    a. Log roll
    b. Recite name and date
    c. Use incentive spirometer
    d. Leg exercises

11. A post-operative client with a leg cast is at risk for developing which of the following complications?

    a. Compartment syndrome
    b. Atelectasis
    c. Pneumonia
    d. Respiratory acidosis

12. While assessing a postoperative client, the nurse checks peripheral circulation. List the steps that the nurse undertakes to do this.

    a. _____
    b. _____
    c. _____
    d. _____

13. On the second postoperative day, a client ambulated with the help of one person and a cane. This level of assistance would be:

    a. Independent
    b. One-person assist
    c. Two-person assist
    d. Independent and device assist

14. Which of the following best describes discharge planning?

    a. Is performed by the admitting nurse only
    b. Begins the day before discharge
    c. Is the health care provider's responsibility to prescribe
    d. Begins the day of admission

15. Which of the following should the nurse do to assess a client's current knowledge base and learning style (select all that apply)?

    a. Provide written materials
    b. Assess the client's level of alertness
    c. Ask questions
    d. Use a variety of learning media
    e. Eliminate interruptions

16. Which of the following should the nurse instruct the client and family regarding postoperative wound care at home?

    a. The dressing must be sterile.
    b. There are no special precautions.
    c. Remove the dressing with clean hands.
    d. Always wear gloves when removing the old dressing.

Alterations in Cardiovascular and Hematological Function

CHAPTER 23

Assessment of Cardiovascular and Hematological Function

1. The nurse realizes that the cellular components of blood are all derived from a:

    a. Red blood cell
    b. White blood cell
    c. Stem cell
    d. Platelet

2. Analysis of the blood provides information about (select all that apply):

    a. Many organ systems
    b. The status of the veins
    c. The status of the arteries
    d. The overall functional status of the body
    e. The status of the heart

3. The production of red blood cells occurs in the _____ _____ and is called _____.

4. Which of the following types of granulocytes is most likely involved in an allergic or asthmatic response?

    a. Neutrophils
    b. Mast cells
    c. Eosinophils
    d. T cells

5. The clotting cascade has two distinct sides. List these sides.

    a. _____
    b. _____

6. The first step of clot formation occurs with which of the following:

    a. Formation of a fibrin clot
    b. Activation of fibrinolysis
    c. Release of Protein C
    d. The platelet

7. Which of the following are antiplatelet medications (select all that apply)?

    a. Lovenox
    b. Aspirin
    c. Ticlid
    d. Activase
    e. ReoPro

8. Which of the following laboratory tests measures a client's extrinsic system or international normalized ratio (INR)?

   a. Prothrombin time
   b. Partial thromboplastin time (PTT)
   c. Thrombin time
   d. Fibrinogen level

9. List the three layers of the heart.

   a. _____
   b. _____
   c. _____

10. Of the following, choose the valves that have two leaflets or cusps (select all that apply):

    a. Pulmonic valve
    b. Tricuspid valve
    c. Aortic valve
    d. Mitral valve

11. The heart receives blood from the coronary arteries that originate from the base of:

    a. The right atrium
    b. The left ventricle
    c. The aorta
    d. The lungs

12. The amount of pressure a heart ventricle must generate to push blood into circulation is called:

    a. Preload
    b. Cardiac output
    c. Afterload
    d. Ejection fraction

13. The diastolic blood pressure reading measures the:

    a. Right atrium at rest
    b. Right ventricle at rest
    c. Left atrium at rest
    d. Left ventricle at rest

14. List the landmarks for conducting a cardiovascular assessment based on the bony structures of the chest.

    a. _____
    b. _____
    c. _____

15. One age-related change in the cardiovascular status is a(n) _____ in the maximum heart rate in response to exercise.

16. Which of the following sources of chest pain is most likely associated with neurological complications?

    a. Aortic dissection
    b. Pericarditis
    c. Pneumothorax
    d. Esophageal rupture

17. Of the following, choose the ones that are considered modifiable risk factors for coronary heart disease (select all that apply).

    a. Age
    b. Race
    c. Smoking
    d. Blood pressure
    e. Cholesterol
    f. Sex

18. The area where the mitral valve sound is best heard is the:

    a. Second intercostal space right of the sternum
    b. Second intercostal space left of the sternum
    c. Third intercostal space left of the sternum
    d. Fifth intercostal space midclavicular line left of the sternum

19. The nurse suspects a client has a fourth heart sound. To better hear this sound, the nurse should use:

    a. The bell of the stethoscope
    b. The diaphragm of the stethoscope
    c. A blood pressure cuff inflated to 200 mm Hg
    d. A Doppler device

20. The nurse is auscultating a client for a diagnosed heart murmur that is moderately loud and can be easily heard. The nurse would document this heart murmur as being which of the following grades?

    a. Grade I
    b. Grade II
    c. Grade III
    d. Grade IV

CHAPTER 24

Coronary Artery Dysfunction: Nursing Management

1. The major modifiable risk factors for coronary artery disease are hyperlipidemia, hypertension, smoking, diabetes, obesity, and a sedentary lifestyle in addition to:

   a. _____

   b. _____

   c. _____

2. A client is found to have a high-density lipoprotein level. This means the client has a high level of:

   a. Bad cholesterol
   b. Blood glucose
   c. Triglycerides
   d. Good cholesterol

3. Which of the following blood pressure readings would categorize a client as having stage 1 hypertension?

   a. 118/68
   b. 122/88
   c. 140/94
   d. 168/102

4. How long will it take a former smoker's risk for developing coronary artery disease to be the same as someone who never has smoked?

   a. Five years
   b. Three years
   c. One year
   d. Six months

5. An atherosclerotic plaque begins with a fatty streak caused by _____ cells.

6. Over many decades a client develops a stable atherosclerotic plaque within one coronary vessel. This means the vessel is:

   a. Less likely to rupture
   b. Functioning normally
   c. Missing a layer of tissue
   d. More likely to rupture

7. List the three clinical manifestations of coronary artery disease.

   a. _____

   b. _____

   c. _____

8. A client who has chest pain only with exercise will most likely have which of the following types of angina?

   a. Prinzmetal's variant
   b. Silent
   c. Stable
   d. Unstable

9. The nurse is assessing a client's chest pain. What do the letters PQRST represent for this assessment?

   P = _____
   Q = _____
   R = _____
   S = _____
   T = _____

10. A client begins to experience chest pain and places a clenched fist over his sternum. This hand placement is called _____ sign.

11. A client with severe right hip arthritis needs a stress test to diagnose coronary artery disease. Which of the following diagnostic tests can be used for this client (select all that apply)?

    a. Electrocardiogram (ECG) exercise stress test
    b. Stress echocardiogram
    c. Pharmacology stress test
    d. Coronary angiography

12. A client is discharged after having coronary artery bypass surgery. Which of the following instructions should the nurse provide to this client?

    a. Apply lotion to the incisional site
    b. Return to work in 2 weeks
    c. Permitted to take hot showers 1 week after surgery
    d. Do not drive for 4 to 6 weeks

13. Which of the following assessment findings would indicate that a client is not tolerating the prescribed beta-blocker?

    a. Shortness of breath and wheezing
    b. Elevated blood perssure
    c. Elevated heart rate
    d. Hot flashes and pruritis

14. Which of the following instructions should the nurse tell a client who is prescribed Zocor?

    a. Can cause hot flashes
    b. Take at bedtime
    c. Call the health care provider if any headaches
    d. Can cause constipation

15. After the placement of a stent in a coronary artery, which of the following medications will be prescribed to prevent vessel restenosis over the long term (select all that apply)?

    a. Heparin
    b. Plavix
    c. ReoPro
    d. Integrilin
    e. Aspirin

16. _____ _____ revascularization, or TMR, is a procedure in which lasers are used to create channels in the left ventricle.

17. The serum blood test that measures myocardial muscle protein in response to myocardial injury is:

    a. Total creatinine kinase (CK)
    b. MB-CK
    c. International normalized ratio (INR)
    d. Troponin level

18. The nurse can follow the mnemonic MONA to provide emergency care to a client with chest pain. What does MONA stand for?
    M = _____
    O = _____
    N = _____
    A = _____

19. When a client or family telephones 911 with chest pain, they will be instructed to have the client chew a(n) _____.

20. A client is participating in cardiac rehabilitation after an acute myocardial infarction. In which phase will this client begin a light exercise program of walking?

    a. I
    b. II
    c. III
    d. IV

Heart Failure and Inflammatory Dysfunction: Nursing Management

1. Which of the following best describes diastolic heart failure?

   a. The ventricles are unable to contract and pump blood.
   b. It is caused by stiff ventricles.
   c. It causes a drop in heart rate.
   d. The heart is unable to relax.

2. Which of the following is a classic symptom of right-sided heart failure?

   a. Peripheral edema
   b. Decreased bowel sounds
   c. Slow heart rate
   d. Increased pedal pulses

3. Which of the following are signs of acute heart failure (select all that apply)?

   a. Muscle spasms
   b. Lung crackles
   c. Pink-tinged sputum
   d. Peripheral edema
   e. Bradycardia

4. Which of the following serum laboratory tests provides the most useful information about the severity of heart failure?

   a. Sodium
   b. Calcium
   c. Potassium
   d. Brain natriuretic peptide (BNP)

5. A client diagnosed with heart failure will benefit from which of the following medications (select all that apply)?

    a. Angiotensin-converting enzyme (ACE) inhibitors
    b. Beta blockers
    c. Calcium channel blockers
    d. Nonsteroidal anti-inflammatory drugs (NSAIDs)
    e. Metformin
    f. Loop diuretics

6. List the four types of cardiomyopathy.

    a. _____
    b. _____
    c. _____
    d. _____

7. The surgical procedure that can be done if medication therapy is ineffective in a client with hypertrophic cardiomyopathy is a(n) _____.

8. Which of the following are the goals of managing a client with arrhythmogenic right-ventricular hypertrophy (select all that apply)?

    a. Minimize symptoms
    b. Prepare for heart transplantation
    c. Plan for emergency cardioversion
    d. Reduce weight
    e. Control arrhythmias

9. Which of the following may be a cause of restrictive cardiomyopathy?

    a. Obesity
    b. Genetic predisposition
    c. History of radiation therapy
    d. Sedentary lifestyle

10. List the three types of carditis.

    a. _____
    b. _____
    c. _____

11. A client is suspected of having acute bacterial endocarditis because of _____ lesions that are flat, painless, red-blue spots on the palms and soles.

12. Which of the following can cause myocarditis (select all that apply)?

    a. Rheumatic heart disease
    b. Parasites
    c. Nitrous oxide
    d. Allergens
    e. Immunosuppressant therapy

13. A client is diagnosed with pericarditis because of the presence of the Beck's triad. List the components of Beck's triad.

    a. _____
    b. _____
    c. _____

14. On auscultating a client's heart sounds, a friction rub is heard. This finding is consistent with:

    a. Endocarditis
    b. Right-sided heart failure
    c. Pericarditis
    d. Systolic heart failure

15. The diagnostic test useful in the diagnosis of cardiac murmurs, stenosis, and cardiac valve diseases is the _____ echocardiography.

16. Which of the following cardiac valve disorders is most often seen in females and might have a genetic component?

    a. Mitral valve prolapse
    b. Aortic regurgitation
    c. Aortic stenosis
    d. Pulmonic regurgitation

17. A client diagnosed with mitral valve regurgitation after an echocardiogram would then be treated similarly to a client diagnosed with:

    a. Pericarditis
    b. Congestive heart failure
    c. Chronic obstructive pulmonary disorder
    d. Hypertension

18. One element of the nursing management of a client diagnosed with aortic regurgitation is:

    a. Weight-reduction techniques
    b. Reporting new symptoms
    c. Teaching antibiotic prophylaxis
    d. Wound care

19. Which of the following medications is contraindicated for a client diagnosed with heart failure?

    a. Loop diuretics
    b. Metformin
    c. Beta blockers
    d. Digoxin

CHAPTER 26

Arrhythmias: Nursing Management

1. Place in order the structures in which an electrical impulse travels through the heart.

   a. Atrioventricular (AV) junction
   b. Bundle of His
   c. AV node
   d. Purkinje fibers
   e. Sinoatrial (SA) node

2. In the event of a malfunctioning SA node, the _____ node serves as an automatic secondary pacemaker in the heart.

3. List the four characteristics of cardiac cells.

   a. _____
   b. _____
   c. _____
   d. _____

4. The nurse notes a wandering baseline on a client who is being cardiac monitored. The nurse should:

   a. Change the wires
   b. Change the batteries
   c. Reapply the electrodes
   d. Obtain a serum potassium level

5. List the two major categories of mechanisms that occur with arrhythmias.

   a. _____
   b. _____

6. A client has a change in heart rate associated with the mechanism of breathing. This arrhythmia is called:

   a. Sinus arrest
   b. Atrial fibrillation
   c. Sinus exit block
   d. Sinus arrhythmia

7. The cardiac arrhythmias most likely to be seen in a client with digoxin toxicity and hypokalemia are (select all that apply):

   a. Atrial flutter
   b. Atrial tachycardia
   c. Atrial fibrillation
   d. Premature junctional complexes

8. A second-degree AV block type 1 is also called the _____ phenomenon or a(n) _____ type 1 second-degree AV block.

9. A client has premature ventricular contractions that all appear the same. These contractions are called:

   a. Multifocal
   b. Multiformed
   c. Uniformed
   d. Nothing

10. List the five Hs of pulseless electrical activity.

   a. _____
   b. _____
   c. _____
   d. _____
   e. _____

11. Which of the following classes of antiarrhythmic medications includes calcium channel blockers?

   a. I
   b. II
   c. III
   d. IV

12. Synchronized cardioversion is delivering an electrical shock to the heart that is synchronized with a client's _____ wave.

13. Implantable cardioverter defibrillators are indicated for which of the following client types?

   a. Sudden cardiac death
   b. Digitalis toxicity
   c. Atrial flutter
   d. Second-degree heart block

14. List the two types of pacemakers.

   a. _____
   b. _____

15. Which of the following methods of pacemakers is best for a client who has a sudden onset of bradycardia?

   a. Temporary
   b. External
   c. Transcardiac
   d. Permanent

16. Which of the following is an indication on electrocardiogram (ECG) monitoring that a client has a pacemaker?

   a. Presence of pacer spikes
   b. Normal sinus rhythm
   c. Prolonged QRS complex
   d. Heart rate 60 beats per minute

17. After delivering two rescue breaths to a client needing cardiopulmonary resuscitation (CPR), the nurse should next:

    a. Call for help
    b. Begin chest compressions
    c. Assess circulation
    d. Give two more breaths

18. What do the letters ABCD in the advanced cardiac life support (ACLS) primary survey represent?

    A = _____
    B = _____
    C = _____
    D = _____

19. The D in the ACLS secondary survey represents:

    a. Defibrillation
    b. Diuretics
    c. Differential diagnosis
    d. Departure

20. Which of the following can be used to help a client with stable tachycardia (select all that apply)?

    a. Carotid massage
    b. Ask the client to cough
    c. Intubate
    d. Begin synchronized cardioversion
    e. Narcotic therapy
    f. Ask the client to bear down

Vascular Dysfunction: Nursing Management

1. A client is diagnosed with thickening of the walls in small arteries. This diagnosis is called:

   a. Atherosclerosis
   b. Diastolic hypertension
   c. Arterial occlusion
   d. Arteriosclerosis

2. Which blood lipid level does smoking affect?

   a. Raises high-density lipoproteins (HDLs)
   b. Lowers HDL
   c. Raises low-density lipoproteins (LDLs)
   d. Lowers LDL

3. Which of the following medications inhibits platelet adhesion and aggregation (select all that apply)?

   a. Lovenox
   b. Orgaran
   c. Aspirin
   d. Trental
   e. Plavix
   f. Ticlid

4. To prevent atherosclerotic plaques, a client and his or her family should be instructed (select all that apply):

   a. How to put on pantyhose
   b. To avoid extremes in temperature
   c. Not to cross the legs
   d. To wear open-toed shoes
   e. To avoid pain medication

5. A(n) _____ originating from the heart is the most common cause of peripheral arterial occlusion.

6. An extremity with an arterial occlusion can be described by the six Ps. List the six Ps.

   a. _____
   b. _____
   c. _____
   d. _____
   e. _____
   f. _____

7. Which of the following nursing diagnoses would be appropriate for a client diagnosed with peripheral arterial occlusive disease?

   a. Knowledge deficit related to self-care and risk prevention
   b. Ineffective peripheral tissue perfusion related to impaired arterial circulation
   c. Pain related to inflammation of the affected extremity
   d. Fear related to actual serious complications

8. A client is diagnosed with an aneurysm that has split the vessel layers and formed a hematoma. This type of aneurysm is called:

   a. False
   b. True
   c. Fusiform
   d. Dissecting

9. Which of the following should be included in the instructions to a client who is discharged after an abdominal aortic aneurysm repair?

   a. Do not lift anything over 15 pounds.
   b. Return to normal activities of daily living.
   c. Drive short distances the first two weeks.
   d. Wound drainage is normal.

10. List the three factors, known as Vitchow's triad, that can lead to venous thrombosis.

    a. _____
    b. _____
    c. _____

11. Dorsiflexing the foot, causing pain in the calf, or a positive _____ sign, is not always indicative of deep vein thrombosis (DVT).

12. The purpose of heparin to treat the diagnosis of DVT is to:

    a. Dissolve the clot
    b. Reduce platelet aggregation
    c. Have the body absorb the clot
    d. Prevent further clot formation

13. Which of the following documentation approaches can be used to ensure that client care documentation is legal and safe?

    a. PAINTER mnemonic
    b. Spreadsheet
    c. Focused
    d. By exception

14. The most severe complication of anticoagulant therapy is _____ from the nose, gums, or other body parts.

15. Which of the following should be instructed as a mandatory restriction in a client diagnosed with Buerger's disease?

    a. Aspirin
    b. Smoking
    c. Use of over-the-counter pain medication
    d. Use of antiembolitic stockings

16. A client is found to have a 20 mm Hg blood pressure difference between the arms. This finding is consistent with:

    a. Buerger's disease
    b. DVT
    c. Subclavian steal syndrome
    d. Raynaud's disease

17. The diagnostic test best used to diagnose Raynaud's disease is:

    a. Echocardiogram
    b. Blood pressure
    c. Serum sodium level
    d. Doppler ultrasound

18. A client with varicose veins should be instructed to (select all that apply):

    a. Avoid strenuous physical activity
    b. Wear constrictive stockings
    c. Increase walking and swimming
    d. Limit intake of green leafy vegetables
    e. Limit protein intake

CHAPTER 28

Hypertension: Nursing Management

1. What else is primary hypertension known as?

   a. _____
   b. _____

2. A 78-year-old male's blood pressure is 168/72 mm Hg. This type of hypertension would be:

   a. Primary
   b. Secondary
   c. Isolated systolic
   d. None of the above. This is normal blood pressure.

3. Which type of body shape is more closely correlated with hypertension?

   a. Apple
   b. Athletic
   c. Slim
   d. Pear

4. The nurse is counseling a client with hypertension on modifiable risk factors. Which of the following contribute to the development of hypertension (select all that apply)?

   a. Intake of three or more alcoholic drinks per day
   b. Age
   c. Race
   d. Intake of caffeine
   e. Cigarette smoking

5. _____ _____ is the difference between systolic and diastolic blood pressures.

6. In a client with dropping blood pressure, which of the following will also decrease to retain sodium, chloride, and water?

   a. Respiratory rate
   b. Heart rate
   c. Cerebral perfusion rate
   d. Glomerular filtration rate (GFR)

7. What is released by the kidneys in response to a drop in GFR?

   a. Antidiuretic hormone
   b. Rennin
   c. Epinephrine
   d. Norepinephrine

8. A client diagnosed with hypertension has no symptoms. This means:

   a. Only the heart is damaged.
   b. There is no end organ damage.
   c. Only the kidneys are damaged.
   d. It was diagnosed before the first symptoms of organ damage.

9. A client has a blood pressure of 130/86 mm Hg. In which of the following classifications of blood pressure would this client be categorized?

   a. Normal
   b. Prehypertensive
   c. Stage 1 hypertensive
   d. Stage 2 hypertensive

10. Which of the following would contribute to an erroneous blood pressure reading (select all that apply)?

    a. Client in pain
    b. Resting for 30 minutes before the reading
    c. Reading
    d. Watching television
    e. Cold examination room
    f. Just finishing a cigarette

11. Diagnostic tests for a client with hypertension provide information about potential
    _____ _____ damage.

12. Which of the following is a treatment recommendation for a client diagnosed with stage I hypertension?

    a. Recheck in two years
    b. Confirm within two months
    c. Lifestyle modifications
    d. Begin medication therapy

13. The eating plan proven to aid in reducing blood pressure while contributing to weight loss is called _____.

14. Which of the following has the highest amount of caffeine?

    a. Decaffeinated espresso
    b. Diet cola
    c. Chocolate milk
    d. Drip coffee

15. List the three components to total fitness.

    a. _____
    b. _____
    c. _____

16. Which of the following is the drug classification of choice to treat isolated systolic hypertension in an older adult?

    a. Vasodilators
    b. Diuretics
    c. Angiotensin-converting enzyme (ACE) inhibitors
    d. ARBs

CHAPTER 29

Hematological Dysfunction: Nursing Management

1. The lymph nodes that are invaded with cancer in Hodgkin's disease contain _____-_____ cells which are surrounded by host inflammatory cells.

2. Which of the following can the nurse do to help a client receiving chemotherapy experiencing gastrointestinal side effects?

   a. Monitor daily temperature
   b. Wear isolation clothing when caring for the client
   c. Provide pain medication
   d. Administer prescribed anti-emetics and encourage fluids

3. The standard treatment for intermediate-grade non-Hodgkin's lymphoma has been _____.

4. List the three main classifications of anemia.

   a. _____
   b. _____
   c. _____

5. The primary treatment for congenital hemolytic anemia is:

   a. Heparin therapy
   b. Splenectomy
   c. Blood transfusion
   d. Platelet transfusion

6. List the four types of sickle cell anemia crisis.

   a. _____
   b. _____
   c. _____
   d. _____

7. Which of the following are manifestations of iron deficiency anemia (select all that apply)?

   a. Spoon-shaped nails
   b. Clubbed fingers
   c. Diarrhea
   d. Cheilosis
   e. Constipation
   f. Pica

8. An elderly client with a vitamin B_{12} deficiency can demonstrate:

    a. Intact extraocular movements
    b. Orientation to person only
    c. Polyneuritis
    d. Bleeding tendency

9. List the two specific types of primary thrombocytopenia.

    a. _____
    b. _____

10. Disseminated intravascular coagulation (DIC) is best described as:

    a. A side effect of vitamin K therapy
    b. A malfunction in clotting that causes hemorrhage
    c. An expected outcome of anticoagulant therapy
    d. A blood disease

11. A client with primary polycythemia may experience _____, or a burning sensation in the fingers and toes.

12. In neutropenia, the white blood cell component affected is the:

    a. Basophil
    b. Macrophage
    c. Neutrophil
    d. Platelet

13. Which of the following should a client with mononucleosis be instructed to do (select all that apply)?

    a. Return to normal activities of daily living
    b. Take frequent rest periods
    c. Avoid over-the-counter pain medication
    d. Restrict vitamin C intake
    e. Avoid strenuous activities

14. Which of the following types of leukemia causes few symptoms and may be discovered during routine blood work?

    a. Chronic lymphocytic
    b. Chronic myeloid
    c. Acute lymphocytic
    d. Acute myeloid

15. A client will be diagnosed with leukemia after a physical examination, blood work, and a(n) _____ _____ biopsy.

16. Which of the following is a client recovering from stem cell transplantation at risk for developing?

    a. Hair loss
    b. Infection
    c. Vitamin B_{12} deficiency
    d. Iron deficiency anemia

17. A client receiving treatment for the diagnosis of acute myeloid leukemia needs postinduction chemotherapy to:

    a. Prevent hair loss
    b. Eliminate leukemic cells from the bone marrow
    c. Prevent neutropenia
    d. Prevent relapse after remission

18. Chronic myelogenous leukemia is associated with the _____ chromosome.

19. A client who works with pesticides is at risk for developing:

    a. Mononucleosis
    b. Aplastic anemia
    c. Multiple myeloma
    d. Vitamin B$_{12}$ deficiency

20. The most common presenting symptom of multiple myeloma is:

    a. Bone pain
    b. Bleeding
    c. Itchy skin
    d. Muscle pain

Alterations in Respiratory Function

CHAPTER 30

Assessment of Respiratory Function

1. Which of the following are considered accessory respiratory muscles (select all that apply)?

   a. Trapezius
   b. Diaphragm
   c. Intercostal
   d. Pectoralis minor
   e. Scalene

2. The portion of ventilatory structures that does not participate in gas exchange is called
   _____ _____.

3. How many generations of airways exist in the entire lower respiratory tract?

   a. 25
   b. 23
   c. 20
   d. 18

4. One of the primary defense mechanisms of the lungs is the mucous blanket, or:

   a. Sneeze reflex
   b. Nose hairs
   c. Cough reflex
   d. Mucociliary escalator

5. If the clinical measure of oxygenation status is PaO_2, then the clinical measure of ventilation status is _____.

6. To determine the degree of hypoxemia, which of the following needs to be done?

   a. Measure pulse oximetry
   b. Count respiratory rate
   c. Measure PaO_2
   d. Check peripheral pulses

7. The oxyhemoglobin dissociation curve is a relationship between the PaO_2 and:

   a. $PaCO_2$
   b. SaO_2
   c. HCO_3
   d. pH

8. List the three mechanisms the body uses to maintain a normal blood pH.

   a. _____
   b. _____
   c. _____

9. The nurse is using the POLK system to interpret arterial blood gases (ABGs). The L in this mnemonic represents:

   a. Legs
   b. Limbs
   c. Limbic system
   d. Lungs

10. List normal arterial blood gas (ABG) levels.

    pH = _____
    PaO_2 = _____
    $PaCO_2$ = _____
    HCO_3 = _____

11. Which of the following is a cause of metabolic acidosis?

    a. Renal failure
    b. Vomiting
    c. Oversedation
    d. Pain

12. Yellow or green sputum can indicate:

    a. Lobar pneumonia
    b. Mitral stenosis
    c. Bronchial infection
    d. Lung abscess

13. The _____ _____ is the amount of air remaining in the lungs at the end of a forced exhalation.

14. The chest shape most commonly seen with chronic emphysema is:

    a. Barrel
    b. Funnel
    c. Pigeon
    d. Kyphosis

15. What do the letters VOPS represent?

    V = _____
    O = _____
    P = _____
    S = _____

16. A client has increased fremitus, which can be caused by (select all that apply):

    a. Pneumonia
    b. Pneumothorax
    c. Pleural tumor
    d. Atelectasis
    e. Pulmonary fibrosis

17. Which of the following adventitious breath sounds is musical?

    a. Pleural friction rub
    b. Rales
    c. Rhonchi
    d. Wheezes

18. The normal vital capacity of an 85-year-old client is:

    a. The same as that of a 30 year old
    b. Thirty percent better than that of a 30 year old
    c. Fifty percent less than that of a 30 year old
    d. Eighty-five percent less than that of a 30 year old

19. The purpose of a ventilation-perfusion lung scan is to diagnose _____
    _____.

20. Which of the following is an important consideration when administering oxygen to a client?

    a. The best way is to use a low-flow system.
    b. It is considered a drug.
    c. All clients need high-flow systems.
    d. Pulse oximetry reading is the only true reflection of arterial oxygenation.

CHAPTER 31

Upper Airway Dysfunction: Nursing Management

1. List the triad of signs that children with allergic rhinitis can exhibit.

   a. _____
   b. _____
   c. _____

2. The nurse is instructing a client with allergic rhinitis on avoidance measures. This instruction should include (select all that apply):

   a. Remove carpeting
   b. Mow the lawn only in the morning
   c. Reduce the use of air conditioning
   d. Maximize the circulation of fresh air in the home
   e. Replace feather or down pillows with synthetics

3. Which of the following medications should be avoided in a client diagnosed with hypertension?

   a. Tavist
   b. Sudafed
   c. Zyrtec
   d. Singular

4. A vaccine to prevent the common cold is difficult to create because:

   a. Everyone would want it.
   b. It is cost prohibitive to create.
   c. There are many different viruses that can cause a cold.
   d. There are other diseases that vaccines are needed for first.

5. Overuse of decongestant nasal sprays can lead to rebound nasal congestion,
   or _____ _____.

6. A client experiencing a sinus infection may complain of (select all that apply):

   a. Neck pain
   b. Unilateral face pain
   c. Headache
   d. Thirst
   e. Pain when chewing
   f. Numb fingers

7. Which of the following antibiotics would be indicated for a client diagnosed with a sinus infection who is allergic to penicillin?

    a. Amoxicillin
    b. Augmentin
    c. Pen V K
    d. Levaquin

8. A 13-year-old client complains of a severe sore throat and pain with swallowing. Which of the following should be done to correctly diagnose this client?

    a. A throat culture
    b. A nasal smear
    c. A sputum sample
    d. A bronchoscopy

9. Which of the following might also be done during a tonsillectomy?

    a. Tubes placed in the middle ear
    b. Repair of deviated nasal septum
    c. Removal of adenoid tissue if inflamed
    d. Irrigation of sinuses

10. A peritonsillar abscess, or _____, is a complication of acute tonsillitis, and the client may speak with a _____ potato voice.

11. A telephone customer service representative is at risk for developing which of the following with a common cold?

    a. Acute laryngitis
    b. Pneumonia
    c. Sinusitis
    d. Peritonsillar abscess

12. List the three types of sleep apnea.

    a. _____
    b. _____
    c. _____

13. Which of the following has been helpful in the treatment of clients diagnosed with obstructive sleep apnea?

    a. Narcotic sleeping aids
    b. Continuous positive airway pressure (CPAP)
    c. Ear plugs
    d. Setting alarm to wake up every two hours

14. The most common cause of epistaxis is _____.

15. What should be included when instructing the parents of a child who experiences frequent nosebleeds (select all that apply)?

    a. Apply petroleum jelly to prevent dryness
    b. Avoid dehumidifiers
    c. Blow the nose frequently
    d. Do not pick the nose
    e. Take aspirin for pain

16. The abdominal thrust technique used to dislodge an item in the throat is called the _____ maneuver.

17. Which of the following increases a person's risk for developing laryngeal cancer?

    a. Stress
    b. Obesity
    c. Smoking and alcohol intake
    d. Hypertension

18. Which of the following procedures for laryngeal cancer will leave a client permanently hoarse but with intact swallowing?

    a. Partial laryngectomy
    b. Supraglottic laryngectomy
    c. Hemilaryngectomy
    d. Total laryngectomy

19. Speech therapy for a client scheduled for a total laryngectomy should begin:

    a. One week after surgery
    b. Three days after surgery
    c. The day of surgery
    d. Before surgery

20. Which of the following should be included in discharge instructions for the client recovering from a laryngectomy?

    a. Need to avoid oral fluids
    b. Time to begin outpatient speech therapy
    c. Reasons to reduce humidity in the home environment
    d. Signs of an infection and when to notify a health care provider

CHAPTER 32

Lower Airway Dysfunction: Nursing Management

1. List the three hallmark symptoms of pulmonary disease for which people seek medical treatment.

   a. _____
   b. _____
   c. _____

2. A client with emphysema is intubated for surgery. Which of the following is the client at risk for developing?

   a. Bacterial pneumonia
   b. Viral pneumonia
   c. Fungal pneumonia
   d. Hospital acquired pneumonia

3. Which of the following are considered extrapulmonary restrictive diseases (select all that apply)?

   a. Lung cancer
   b. Pneumonia
   c. Flail chest
   d. Rib fractures
   e. Asthma
   f. Pneumothorax

4. A client who is HIV negative has been exposed to tuberculosis. Which of the following medication regimens would be appropriate for this client?

   a. Isoniazid (INH) for 12 months
   b. INH for 6 months
   c. Rifampin
   d. Ethambutol

5. The four most common pulmonary fungal infections include coccidioidomycosis and what other three infections?

   a. _____
   b. _____
   c. _____

6. Which of the following are side effects of oral antifungal medications (select all that apply)?

    a. Diarrhea
    b. Headache
    c. Rash
    d. Constipation
    e. Vertigo
    f. Secondary herpes simplex infection

7. List the three types of bronchiectasis.

    a. _____
    b. _____
    c. _____

8. Which of the following medications are indicated for a client with a lung abscess who is allergic to penicillin?

    a. Metronidazole
    b. Amoxicillin
    c. Gentamycin
    d. Clindamycin

9. According to the National Comprehensive Caner Network, most types of cancers are staged according to TNM. What does TNM stand for?

    T = _____
    N = _____
    M = _____

10. Which of the following types of diets can be recommended for a client receiving treatment for lung cancer?

    a. DASH
    b. C
    c. Liquid
    d. 1,800 calorie

11. List the four types of pneumothorax.

    a. _____
    b. _____
    c. _____

12. Which of the following aids in the diagnosis of pneumothorax?

    a. Abdominal flat plate
    b. Serum sodium level
    c. Arterial blood gas
    d. Sputum sample

13. Which of the following should be done if a client's chest tube becomes dislodged?

    a. Apply Vaseline gauze and tape on all four sides
    b. Apply Vaseline gauze and tape on three sides
    c. Apply Vaseline gauze and tape on two sides
    d. Apply Vaseline gauze and tape on one side

14. The nurse, planning the care for a client with rib fractures, will include interventions to prevent which of the following complications from occurring? (Select all that apply.)

    a. Pulmonary hypertension
    b. Pneumonia
    c. Cor pulmonale
    d. Heart failure
    e. Atelectasis

15. List the two main types of pulmonary artery hypertension.

    a. _____
    b. _____

16. Which of the following diseases does pulmonary artery hypertension mimic (select all that apply)?

    a. Congestive heart failure
    b. Pneumonia
    c. Chronic obstructive pulmonary disorder
    d. Irritable bowel syndrome
    e. Atrial fibrillation

17. A complete blood count finding in a client diagnosed with cor pulmonale would be:

    a. Low white blood cell count
    b. Low platelets
    c. Elevated basophils
    d. Polycythemia

18. Which of the following would be included as treatment for a client diagnosed with cor pulmonale (select all that apply)?

    a. Intravenous (IV) Lasix
    b. Walk six times a day for 30 minutes each time
    c. Limit meals to two per day
    d. Cough and do deep breathing exercises every two hours
    e. Oxygen, 6 liters via face mask

Obstructive Pulmonary Disease: Nursing Management

1. Which of the following anatomical shapes is typically seen in a client diagnosed with chronic obstructive pulmonary disorder (COPD)?

   a. Pigeon
   b. Kyphosis
   c. Barrel
   d. Scoliosis

2. The diseases emphysema and chronic bronchitis have been called pink _____ and blue _____.

3. Choose all that are characteristics of COPD:

   a. Sputum production
   b. Joint pain
   c. Gastric distress
   d. Dyspnea on exertion
   e. Cough

4. At which stage of COPD does a client's lung function still measure as normal?

   a. 0
   b. I
   c. II
   d. III

5. The diagnostic test least likely to assist in the diagnoses of COPD is:

   a. Chest X-ray
   b. Sputum culture
   c. Computed tomography (CT) scan
   d. Electrocardiogram (ECG)

6. A client has not smoked for 24 hours. Which of the following physiological conditions has improved?

   a. Lung function by 30 percent
   b. Oxygen levels near normal
   c. Decreased risk for myocardial infarction
   d. Circulation

7. Which of the following increases a client's risk of developing complications from the flu? (Select all that apply.)

   a. Age 70
   b. Diagnosis of heart failure
   c. Exercises 3 times each week for 30 minutes
   d. Treatment for type 2 diabetes mellitus for 5 years
   e. Current BMI 24

8. The mucous clearing drug of choice for a client diagnosed with COPD is:

   a. Expectorant
   b. Mucolytic
   c. Inhaled corticosteroid
   d. Water

9. The type of breathing technique that decreases air trapped in the lungs, promotes relaxation, and can increase an oxygen saturation level to at least 93 percent is called:

   a. Pursed lip
   b. Huff
   c. Diaphragmatic
   d. Pant

10. The client who has an acute onset of asthma when in the presence of dogs is reacting to which of the following categories of asthmatic triggers?

    a. Air pollution
    b. Environmental
    c. Pharmacology
    d. Exercise

11. The client who experiences asthma symptoms at night about every two weeks would be classified as having which level of asthma severity?

    a. Step 1
    b. Step 2
    c. Step 3
    d. Step 4

12. Pulmonary function spirometry tests for a person diagnosed with asthma should be conducted (select all that apply):

    a. Every week
    b. During the first assessment
    c. Every month
    d. Every one to two years
    e. Once to diagnose

13. What do the following colors used in the asthma action plan signify?

    Green = _____
    Yellow = _____
    Red = _____

14. The preferred medication regimen for a client diagnosed with step 2, mild, persistent asthma is:

    a. High dose inhaled corticosteroid
    b. Low dose inhaled corticosteroid
    c. Nothing
    d. Short-acting bronchodilator

15. Choose the goals of asthma treatment (select all that apply):

    a. Miss only five days of work or school per month
    b. Minimal or no symptoms during the day or night
    c. Near normal pulmonary function
    d. Headaches at bedtime only
    e. Bad taste in mouth present
    f. No side effects from medication

16. _____ is a condition that can occur as a result of increased air pressure in the lungs.

17. In a client diagnosed with cystic fibrosis, the pilocarpine iontophoresis sweat test will show:

    a. Normal
    b. Low sodium level
    c. High sodium level
    d. Low magnesium level

18. The only definitive treatment for advanced cystic fibrosis is _____
    _____.

19. The best-studied antibiotic used to treat lower respiratory tract infections in clients diagnosed with cystic fibrosis is:

    a. Tobramycin
    b. Penicillin
    c. Amoxicillin
    d. Augmentin

7

Alterations in Neurological Function

Assessment of Neurological Function

1. List two cell types that compose the entire nervous system.

   a. _____
   b. _____

2. Myelinated axons are called:

   a. Gray matter
   b. Dendrites
   c. Cell bodies
   d. White matter

3. Choose the components needed for nerve impulse transmission (select all that apply):

   a. Gray matter
   b. Presynaptic terminal
   c. Synaptic cleft
   d. White matter
   e. Receptor site
   f. Dendrite

4. Into which of the following classifications of neurotransmitters would endorphins be placed?

   a. Amines
   b. Catecholamines
   c. Amino acids
   d. Polypeptides

5. Which of the following types of neuroglial cells plays a scavenger role?

   a. Oligodendroglia
   b. Microglia
   c. Ependymal
   d. Astrocytes

6. List the central nervous system's (CNS) two major divisions.

   a. _____
   b. _____

7. Identify the number of bones within each segment of the vertebral column:

   Cervical = _____

   Thoracic = _____

   Lumbar = _____

   Sacral = _____

   Coccygeal = _____

8. The thick band of white fibers that allows the two brain hemispheres to communicate would be:

   a. Gray matter
   b. White matter
   c. Meninges
   d. Corpus callosum

9. The part of the CNS that controls voluntary muscle movement and equilibrium would be the:

   a. Cerebellum
   b. Brainstem
   c. Diencephalon
   d. Frontal lobes

10. Which of the following provide blood to the cerebral tissue (select all that apply)?

    a. Dural sinuses
    b. Vertebral arteries
    c. Basilar arteries
    d. Jugular veins
    e. Internal carotid arteries

11. Name the two cranial nerves that have parasympathetic components.

    a. _____
    b. _____

12. Which of the following are characteristics of the parasympathetic system (select all that apply)?

    a. Rest and repair
    b. Decreased heart rate
    c. Dilated pupils
    d. General housekeeping
    e. Fight or flight

13. List the three categories assessed with the Glasgow coma scale.

    a. _____
    b. _____
    c. _____

14. To assess the spinal accessory nerve (CN XI), the nurse could ask the client to:

    a. Grasp hands
    b. Shrug shoulders
    c. Make a fist
    d. Press down on the gas pedal

15. The nurse finds that one muscle group of a client has active movement against gravity, but the nurse is able to overcome the client's muscle resistance. The nurse would grade this muscle strength as:

    a. Grade 0
    b. Grade 2
    c. Grade 4
    d. Grade 5

16. A client is unable to perform rapid alternating movements with one muscle group. This finding is called:

    a. Dysdiadochokinesia
    b. Dyssynergy
    c. Dysmetria
    d. Ataxia

17. The nurse finds a client's deep tendon reflexes to be normal or average. This finding is rated as:

    a. 4+
    b. 3+
    c. 2+
    d. 1+

18. The _____ _____ is the most common method for obtaining cerebrospinal fluid.

19. Which of the following diagnostic tests would be contraindicated for a client with metal plates from a spinal fusion?

    a. Magnetic resonance imaging (MRI)
    b. Computed tomography (CT) scan
    c. Lumbar puncture
    d. Spinal X-rays

20. Which of the following diagnostic tests measures the electrical activity of the peripheral nerves by testing muscle activity?

    a. EP
    b. Electroencephalogram (EEG)
    c. Ultrasound
    d. Electromyography (EMG)

CHAPTER 35

Dysfunction of the Brain: Nursing Management

1. List the two main types of stroke.

   a. _____
   b. _____

2. Which of the following are modifiable risk factors for a stroke (select all that apply)?

   a. Family history
   b. Atrial fibrillation
   c. Age
   d. Drug use
   e. Hypertension
   f. Sex

3. Which of the following is the best outcome for stroke management?

   a. Prevention
   b. Only go to a stroke hospital for care
   c. Take aspirin every day
   d. Avoid obesity

4. Which of the following is the drug of choice for a client diagnosed with an ischemic stroke?

   a. Vitamin K
   b. Heparin
   c. Coumadin
   d. Tissue plasminogen activator (tPA)

5. Which of the following should be included in the care of a client post tPA (select all that apply)?

   a. Neurological checks every 15 minutes for two hours
   b. Place nasogastric tube for medications
   c. Provide aspirin 81 mg by mouth (PO) every morning
   d. No intravenous (IV) catheter placement
   e. Begin Coumadin 5 mp PO every evening

6. Which of the following nursing diagnoses would be appropriate for the family providing care at home to a client with a stroke?

   a. Coping
   b. Risk for caregiver role strain
   c. Impaired verbal communication
   d. Risk for disturbed self-esteem

7. The major cause of traumatic brain injury is _____ _____ accidents.

8. An injury that causes brain damage as a result of an external force is called:

   a. Open injury
   b. Secondary injury
   c. Traumatic brain injury
   d. Closed injury

9. List the three levels of brain injury.

   a. _____
   b. _____
   c. _____

10. A brain-injured client is awakened, opens his eyes, and responds to pain; however, he is not aware of his surroundings. The status of this patient is:

    a. Vegetative state
    b. Locked-in syndrome
    c. Coma
    d. Minimally responsive state

11. Most head-injury clients who sustain a brain injury will present with symptoms in which of the following categories (select all that apply)?

    a. Behavioral
    b. Socioeconomic
    c. Environmental
    d. Cognitive
    e. Physical

12. Which of the following neurological bleeds can appear two weeks after the initial injury and be mistaken for a stroke?

    a. Acute subdural hematoma
    b. Subacute subdural hematoma
    c. Epidural hematoma
    d. Subarachnoid hemorrhage

13. The purpose of a(n) _____ pressure monitoring device is to prevent a secondary brain injury after trauma to the head.

14. When planning care for a client having a craniotomy to remove a brain tumor, the nurse should include interventions to address which of the following most frequent complications?

    a. Pneumonia
    b. Hemorrhage
    c. Urinary tract infection
    d. Venous thromboembolism

15. The most common type of brain tumor is a(n) _____.

16. The tests most commonly used to diagnose a brain tumor are (select all that apply):

    a. Magnetic resonance imaging (MRI)
    b. Doppler studies
    c. White blood cell (WBC) count
    d. Skull X-rays
    e. Computed tomography (CT) scan

17. List the three main types of treatment for a client with a brain tumor.

    a. _____
    b. _____
    c. _____

18. A medication that helps chemotherapeutic agents cross the blood-brain barrier is:

    a. Mannitol
    b. Lasix
    c. Amoxicillin
    d. Augmentin

19. The type of aphasia in which a client knows what they want to say but cannot get the words to form is called:

    a. Receptive
    b. Communicative
    c. Expressive
    d. Global

Dysfunction of the Spinal Cord and Peripheral Nervous System: Nursing Management

1. The outer layers of the spinal cord are made up of:

   a. Cerebral spinal fluid
   b. White matter
   c. Tendons
   d. Gray matter

2. Damage to upper motor neurons will result in:

   a. Flaccid paralysis
   b. Increased cerebral spinal fluid
   c. Spasticity
   d. Hemiparesis

3. Hemisection of the spinal cord will lead to _____ _____ syndrome.

4. The most common spinal cord injuries are (select all that apply):

   a. T 11 to 12
   b. C 4 to 6
   c. L 5 to S 1
   d. T 1 to 2
   e. C 1 to 2

5. Which of the following scales categorizes the degree of incomplete spinal cord injury and expectations for functioning?

   a. Glasgow coma scale
   b. University of Alabama (UAB)
   c. MOPS
   d. American Spinal Injury Association (ASIA)

6. The standard of care used to stabilize fractured cervical vertebra is the _____ traction.

7. The medication of choice for a client who sustained a spinal cord injury less than four hours ago is:

   a. Coumadin
   b. Methylprednisolone
   c. Heparin
   d. Tissue plasminogen activator (tPA)

8. Which of the following are tested to evaluate the resolution of spinal shock (select all that apply)?

   a. Babinski reflex
   b. Respiratory rate
   c. Electrocardiogram (ECG)
   d. Cremasteric reflex
   e. Electroencephalogram (EEG)
   f. Arterial blood gas (ABG)

9. A client with a spinal cord injury has a blood pressure of 210/120 mm Hg. This could indicate _____ _____.

10. Which of the following interventions is appropriate during the rehabilitation of a client with paraplegia and bladder dysfunction?

    a. Teach self-catheterization
    b. Place indwelling catheter
    c. Restrict fluids
    d. Advise to expect a future kidney stone

11. To prevent the onset of decubitus ulcers in a client recovering from a spinal cord injury, which of the following should the nurse do?

    a. Limit position changes
    b. Use a donut on the seat of the wheelchair
    c. Create and adhere to a turning schedule
    d. Perform passive range of motion exercises daily

12. A client recovering from a spinal cord injury states, "I think I can still work if I'm in a wheelchair." This is demonstrating which stage of grief for clients with spinal cord injuries?

    a. Shock
    b. Denial
    c. Anger
    d. Adjustment

13. The majority of spinal cord tumors are _____, or located outside of the spinal cord.

14. Which of the following peripheral nerve disorders is being investigated for an association for occurrence after a vaccination, surgical procedure, or stressful event?

    a. Bell's palsy
    b. Trigeminal neuralgia
    c. Mèniére's disease
    d. Guillain-Barré syndrome

15. List the three divisions of the trigeminal nerve.

    a. _____
    b. _____
    c. _____

16. The medication most commonly used to treat trigeminal neuralgia is:

   a. Baclofen
   b. Tegretol
   c. Capsaicin
   d. Gabapentin

17. The most common cause of facial paralysis is _____ _____.

18. Which of the following treatments would be used first to treat carpal tunnel syndrome?

   a. Corticosteroid injections
   b. Surgery
   c. Nerve block
   d. Hand and wrist splints

19. A client diagnosed with carpal tunnel syndrome will have worse pain:

   a. In the morning
   b. After eating
   c. When using warm water
   d. At night

CHAPTER 37

Degenerative Neurological Dysfunction: Nursing Management

1. The most common form of chronic pain is:

   a. Headache
   b. Backache
   c. Wrist ache
   d. Toothache

2. List the three types of primary headache.

   a. _____
   b. _____
   c. _____

3. The beta blocker that can be prescribed to treat a tension headache is:

   a. Calan
   b. Imitrex
   c. Stadol
   d. Inderal

4. Sensitivities common in clients diagnosed with migraine headaches include: (Select all that apply.)

   a. Osmophobia
   b. Agoraphobia
   c. Claustrophobia
   d. Phonophobia
   e. Arachnophobia
   f. Photophobia

5. A client diagnosed with migraine headaches should be instructed to avoid:

   a. Meat
   b. Red wine
   c. Yogurt
   d. Chicken

6. Characteristics of cluster headaches include (select all that apply):

   a. Nausea
   b. Pain behind one eye
   c. Rhinorrhea
   d. Vomiting
   e. Photophobia

7. List the four phases of a seizure.

   a. _____
   b. _____
   c. _____
   d. _____

8. Todd's paralysis can occur in which phase of a seizure?

   a. Aural
   b. Ictal
   c. Prodromal
   d. Postictal

9. Which type of seizure causes a client to suddenly lose muscle control to the legs, leading to falls?

   a. Absence
   b. Atonic
   c. Myoclonic
   d. Partial

10. First-line drugs used to treat seizures are (select all that apply):

    a. Ativan
    b. Tegretol
    c. Klonopin
    d. Mysoline
    e. Versed
    f. Dilantin

11. The most common category and form of multiple sclerosis is:

    a. Primary progressive
    b. Progressive-relapsing
    c. Relapsing-remitting
    d. Secondary progressive

12. Which of the following medications is helpful to treat neuropathic pain in a client diagnosed with multiple sclerosis?

    a. Neurontin
    b. Prozac
    c. Ditropan
    d. Urecholine

13. Using the mnemonic TRAP, identify major clinical manifestations of Parkinson's disease.

    T = _____
    R = _____
    A = _____
    P = _____

14. The primary goal of Parkinson's disease management is to:

    a. Achieve a cure
    b. Prevent functional disability
    c. Avoid skin breakdown
    d. Maintain self-feeding ability

15. A medication useful in improving cognition for a client diagnosed with Alzheimer's disease is:

    a. Luvox
    b. Zoloft
    c. Aricept
    d. Haldol

16. The diagnostic test used to see if a client has improvement in manifestations of myasthenia gravis is:

    a. Tensilon test
    b. Serum assay
    c. Electromyography (EMG)
    d. Computed tomography (CT) scan

17. The typical cause of death in clients diagnosed with amyotrophic lateral sclerosis is:

    a. Cardiac arrest
    b. Respiratory arrest
    c. Urinary tract infection
    d. Deep vein thrombosis

18. A client diagnosed with amyotrophic lateral sclerosis may develop _____ _____ syndrome because of progressive paralysis.

19. The primary cause of Huntington's chorea is:

    a. Exposure to pesticides
    b. Elevated lipid levels
    c. No known cause
    d. Genetic

Alterations in Sensory Function

Assessment of Sensory Function

1. The cranial nerve responsible for transmitting visual stimuli to the brain for interpretation is:

   a. I
   b. II
   c. III
   d. IV

2. The cranial nerves responsible for extraocular movements are (select all that apply):

   a. II
   b. III
   c. IV
   d. V
   e. VI

3. In which internal eye structure is the cornea found?

   a. Outer
   b. Middle
   c. Inner
   d. Conjunctiva

4. Stimulation of cranial nerve V causes the _____ reflex, or a protective eye blink.

5. List the four sets of blood vessels that supply the optic disc.

   a. _____
   b. _____
   c. _____
   d. _____

6. An eye examination should begin with:

   a. Palpation of extraocular structures
   b. Ophthalmoscopic examination
   c. Visual field testing
   d. Visual acuity

7. The chart used to assess color vision is:

   a. Snellen's chart
   b. Rosenbaum chart
   c. Ishihara chart
   d. OLDCART chart

8. List the eye responses that are tested by shining a penlight into one eye.

   a. _____
   b. _____

9. The most common complaints of long-term ear problems are because of (select all that apply):

   a. Hearing loss
   b. Pain
   c. Discharge
   d. Vertigo
   e. Tinnitus

10. _____is defined as liquid discharge or drainage from the ear.

11. When using the voice-whisper test to assess hearing, a normal finding is that the client is able to repeat words whispered at a distance of:

   a. 6 inches
   b. 12 inches
   c. 18 inches
   d. 24 inches

12. Diagnostic tests done to assess conductive or sensorineural hearing loss are (select all that apply):

   a. Romberg
   b. Weber
   c. Rinne
   d. Ultrasound
   e. Electromyographs (EMGs)

13. When palpating the ear, a normal exam finding is:

   a. Pain
   b. Crepitus
   c. Discharge
   d. No client response

14. To straighten the ear canal before introducing an otoscope in an adult's ear, the nurse should:

   a. Pull the ear down and back
   b. Tug the pinna forward
   c. Pull the ear up and back
   d. Bend the ear lobe back

15. Which of the following would be considered abnormal findings from an otoscopic examination (select all that apply)?

   a. Thin cerumen
   b. White plaques
   c. Peripheral blood vessels
   d. Air bubbles
   e. Moveable tympanic membrane
   f. Blood

CHAPTER 39

Visual Dysfunction: Nursing Management

1. List the three main ocular movement dysfunctions.

    a. _____

    b. _____

    c. _____

2. Which of the following is the term for an eye that deviates outward?

    a. Exotropia
    b. Diplopia
    c. Amblyopia
    d. Estropia

3. _____ is an involuntary rhythmic movement of the eyes in a back-and-forth or cyclical movement.

4. Ocular muscle paralysis can be caused by (select all that apply):

    a. Jugular vein distention
    b. Diabetes mellitus
    c. Right heart failure
    d. Myasthenia gravis
    e. Fatigue
    f. Trauma

5. Treatment of ocular motor problems begins with:

    a. Surgery
    b. Oral medications
    c. Correction of refractive errors
    d. Nothing

6. List the risks for developing cataracts.

    a. _____

    b. _____

    c. _____

    d. _____

7. Which of the following are symptoms of cataracts (select all that apply)?

    a. Cloudy vision
    b. Faded colors
    c. Eye tearing
    d. Photophobia
    e. Poor blink response

8. The type of vision that results when an intraocular lens cannot be inserted after cataract surgery is:

    a. Diplopia
    b. Color blindness
    c. Aphakic
    d. Homonymous hemianopsia

9. The eye disorder that causes a sudden headache, blurred vision, and eye pain, which results in increased intraocular pressure, is _____ _____ glaucoma.

10. The purpose of surgery for glaucoma is to:

    a. Stop the progression of the disease
    b. Implant a lens
    c. Prevent cataracts
    d. Cure the disease

11. The medication of choice to treat glaucoma is:

    a. Xanax
    b. Xalatan
    c. Xeloda
    d. Xenical

12. One treatment for a detached retina is to freeze the tear area, or perform_____.

13. The most common type of age-related macular degeneration is:

    a. Refractory
    b. Neovascular
    c. Atrophic
    d. Idiopathic

14. List the three types of corneal disorders.

    a. _____
    b. _____
    c. _____

15. The primary treatment for a client diagnosed with keratoconus is:

    a. Photocoagulation surgery
    b. Soft contact lenses
    c. Cataract removal
    d. Rigid contact lenses

16. Which of the following describes nearsightedness?

    a. Myopia
    b. Astigmatism
    c. Hyperopia
    d. Nystagmus

17. Overall management of inflammatory and infectious eye conditions includes (select all that apply):

    a. Eye patches
    b. Corrective lenses
    c. Antibiotic ointment
    d. Hard contact lenses
    e. Warm, moist compresses

18. Which of the following is an inflammation of the eyelashes causing a sticky exudate?

    a. Keratitis
    b. Blepharitis
    c. Dry eye syndrome
    d. Conjunctivitis

19. Legal blindness is defined as:

    a. 5/100 on the Snellen chart
    b. 10/100 on the Snellen chart
    c. 1/10 on the Snellen chart
    d. 20/200 on the Snellen chart

20. The most common cause of blindness is:

    a. Glaucoma
    b. Macular degeneration
    c. Cataracts
    d. Diabetic retinopathy

CHAPTER 40

Auditory Dysfunction: Nursing Management

1. Which of the following can lead to an auditory dysfunction (select all that apply)?

   a. Diet low in fat
   b. Furosemide therapy
   c. Loud music
   d. Fluid restriction
   e. Excessive use of power tools

2. The organ of Corti is located within the _____ ear.

3. A client is found to require 41 to 55 decibels to hear. This degree of hearing impairment is:

   a. Normal hearing
   b. Slight hearing loss
   c. Mild hearing impairment
   d. Moderate hearing impairment

4. List the three ways to classify auditory dysfunction.

   a. _____
   b. _____
   c. _____

5. Which of the following are characteristics of conductive hearing loss (select all that apply)?

   a. Better hearing in noisy situations
   b. Always caused by an inner ear infection
   c. Has to speak in a louder voice
   d. Can be caused by otosclerosis
   e. Has to speak in a softer voice

6. Management during the acute phase of Mèniére's disease would involve:

   a. Antihistamines
   b. No activity restrictions
   c. Increased sodium intake
   d. Restriction of fluids

7. One symptom of labyrinthitis is:

   a. Nystagmus
   b. Vertigo
   c. Diplopia
   d. Otalgia

8. The most common ear disorder associated with aging is _____.

9. If left untreated, chronic otitis media can lead to:

   a. Multiple sclerosis
   b. Trigeminal neuralgia
   c. Mastoiditis
   d. Nothing

10. A client's tympanometry reading is a flat line. This means:

    a. Normal functioning
    b. The nurse did not do the test correctly.
    c. The client is elderly.
    d. Either a perforation or an obstruction exists.

11. Which of the following should the nurse instruct a client diagnosed with otitis externa to do (select all that apply)?

    a. Use ear plugs
    b. Avoid water sports
    c. No restrictions
    d. Dry the external canal after bathing
    e. Use castor oil to keep the canal moist

12. With otitis media, the tympanic membrane can appear reddish-blue in color. This is also called a positive _____ sign.

13. Which of the following should the nurse instruct a client recovering from a stapedectomy?

    a. Limit the intake of milk products
    b. No limits on activity
    c. Stay on bedrest for 1 week
    d. Avoid sudden head movement

14. A client diagnosed with otosclerosis could benefit from a:

    a. Mastoidectomy
    b. Stapedectomy
    c. Myringotomy
    d. Myringoplasty

15. The surgical procedure found to help with sensorineural hearing loss is a (n) _____ implant.

16. The best approach to treating a hearing disorder is:

    a. To do nothing
    b. Prevention
    c. Have monthly hearing tests
    d. Decrease nicotine intake by half

17. Which of the following should be addressed with a client who has a hearing disorder (select all that apply)?

    a. Ways to avoid the use of a hearing aid
    b. Ways to prevent social isolation
    c. Nothing different
    d. Where to go to learn sign language
    e. Personal safety

18. List the two types of hearing aids.

    a. _____
    b. _____

Alterations in Immunological Function

CHAPTER 41

Assessment of Immunological Function

1. List the three barriers that are considered to be part of the innate immune system.

   a. _____
   b. _____
   c. _____

2. Which of the following is the term used to describe a fully mature monocyte?

   a. Neutrophil
   b. Band cell
   c. Basophil
   d. Macrophage

3. The immunity present at birth is called:

   a. Innate
   b. Adaptive
   c. Specific
   d. Humoral mediated

4. _____ immunity refers to immunity mediated by T lymphocytes.

5. Which of the following describes B lymphocytes (select all that apply)?

   a. Function is poorly understood
   b. Become plasma cells
   c. Mature in the thymus gland
   d. Complex development
   e. Mature in the bone marrow

6. List the four basic functions of antibodies.

   a. _____
   b. _____
   c. _____
   d. _____

7. Interferons are a class of _____ because they interfere with viral replication in uninfected cells.

8. One vital characteristic of the adaptive immune system is:

    a. Clot formation
    b. Renin-angiotensin system
    c. Memory
    d. Sodium-potassium balance

9. Which of the following could be seen in an elderly client diagnosed with an infectious process?

    a. Elevated temperature
    b. Normal response to infections
    c. Evidence body is fighting the infection
    d. Nothing

10. Which of the following can occur if a client has received the Bacillus-Guerin vaccine against tuberculosis?

    a. Nothing
    b. False positive with a purified-protein derivative (PPD) skin test
    c. Active tuberculosis with symptoms
    d. Active disease without symptoms

11. A client who has a history of gastric distress with use of nonsteroidal anti-inflammatory drugs (NSAIDs) should identify this response as a(n):

    a. Allergy
    b. Normal response
    c. Sign the medication dose is too weak
    d. Adverse reaction

12. Which of the following could indicate impaired immune function (select all that apply)?

    a. Red blood cell count within normal limits
    b. Present pedal pulses
    c. Rhinitis
    d. Night sweats
    e. Diarrhea

13. Which of the following skin assessment findings would be seen in a client diagnosed with immune dysfunction?

    a. Petechia
    b. Local maculopapular rash
    c. Dermographism
    d. Bruises
    e. Venous stasis ulcers
    f. Malar rash

14. The most common cause of neutropenia is:

    a. Infection
    b. Bleeding
    c. Diabetes mellitus
    d. Hypertension

15. Which diagnostic tests can be used to determine if a disease is caused by inflammation? (Select all that apply.)

    a. Erythrocyte sedimentation rate
    b. Serum sodium
    c. Partial prothrombin time (PTT)
    d. C-Reactive protein
    e. Total complement

16. Which of the following can be found in healthy older adults? (Select all that apply.)
    a. Elevated neutrophils
    b. Antinuclear antibodies (ANA)
    c. Minimal monocytes
    d. Elevated C-Reactive protein
    e. Rheumatoid factor (RF)

17. The PPD test to screen for tuberculosis is considered a(n) _____ test.

CHAPTER 42

Immunodeficiency and HIV Infection/AIDS: Nursing Management

1. A pregnant client who is HIV positive should be counseled that the baby could be exposed to the virus during _____ _____ and _____.

2. Which of the following criteria are used to establish the diagnosis of AIDS (select all that apply)?

   a. CD4+ below 200 cells/mcgLiter
   b. Development of opportunistic cancer
   c. Presence of end-stage renal disease
   d. Elevated red blood cell count
   e. Wasting syndrome

3. Which of the following opportunistic health problems has become less common in the client diagnosed with AIDS receiving HAART medication therapy?

   a. Shingles
   b. Spinal stenosis
   c. Kaposi's sarcoma
   d. Osteoarthritis

4. Which of the following diagnostic tests can be used to confirm a positive ELISA test for a client?

   a. Sedimentation rate
   b. Western blot test
   c. Platelet count
   d. Red blood cell count

5. A client diagnosed with HIV does not want the hospital chaplain to talk with him in the hospital. The nursing diagnosis appropriate for this patient is:

   a. Decisional conflict
   b. Chronic low self-esteem
   c. Interrupted family processes
   d. Spiritual distress

6. The nurse is instructing a client diagnosed with HIV and the client's family about medication therapy. For which of the following symptoms should the nurse instruct the patient and family to contact the health care provider (select all that apply)?

   a. Diarrhea
   b. Chest pain
   c. Vomiting
   d. Change in vision
   e. Headache
   f. Rash

7. A client newly diagnosed with HIV is prescribed HAART therapy. The nurse realizes HAART means _____.

8. A client who had a kidney transplant four months ago is admitted with signs of organ rejection. The nurse realizes this patient is demonstrating:

   a. Acute rejection
   b. Chronic graft-versus-host (GVH) disease
   c. A normal response to the body accepting the new organ
   d. A side effect of the medication

9. A client admitted with rheumatoid arthritis has severe joint deformity. The nurse realizes this deformity occurs in four phases. List the four phases.

   a. _____
   b. _____
   c. _____
   d. _____

10. A client diagnosed with rheumatoid arthritis is complaining of problems with her eyes. The nurse realizes this patient is experiencing:

    a. Sjögren's syndrome
    b. Early cataract formation
    c. Retinitis
    d. Sty formation

11. During an assessment, the nurse suspects a client is experiencing undiagnosed rheumatoid arthritis. Which of the following findings would support this nurse's assumption (select all that apply)?

    a. Morning stiffness for about 30 minutes
    b. Pain and stiffness of both hand and wrist joints
    c. Palpable nodules over bony prominences
    d. Pain in the right knee only
    e. Pain in the left ankle only

12. The nurse is planning care for a client diagnosed with rheumatoid arthritis. Which of the following would be appropriate nursing outcomes classifications (NOCs) for the diagnosis of activity intolerance (select all that apply)?

    a. Mobility
    b. Self-care activities of daily living
    c. Activity tolerance
    d. Pain control
    e. Endurance
    f. Energy conservation

13. During the assessment of a client diagnosed with rheumatoid arthritis, the nurse learns the client is prescribed Indocin. Which of the following questions should the nurse ask this client?

    a. Are you avoiding alcohol consumption?
    b. When was your last blood test for liver function?
    c. When was your last chest X-ray?
    d. Are you taking anything to protect your stomach?

14. A client is admitted with total body pain and a strange red rash on the face. The nurse realizes this client might be experiencing:

    a. Acute onset of rheumatoid arthritis
    b. Systemic lupus erythematosus (SLE)
    c. Sjögren's syndrome
    d. Scleroderma

15. A client diagnosed with SLE is being discharged. Which of the following should the nurse include in the discharge instructions for this client (select all that apply)?

    a. Tips to reduce calories in the diet
    b. Reminder to avoid sun exposure
    c. Ways to ensure optimal skin care
    d. Telephone number of the local SLE support group
    e. Need to adhere to prescribed medication regime

16. The nurse is assessing a client diagnosed with scleroderma and will use the acronym CREST. This acronym means:

    C = _____
    R = _____
    E = _____
    S = _____
    T = _____

Allergic Dysfunction: Nursing Management

1. List the three categories of immune responses.

   a. _____

   b. _____

   c. _____

2. Which of the following Rs within the immune response produces antibodies in the presence of non-self-invaders?

   a. Recognize
   b. Respond
   c. Remember
   d. Regulate

3. What type of hypersensitivity reaction is a blood transfusion reaction categorized as?

   a. Anaphylactic
   b. Cytotoxic
   c. Immune complex
   d. Delayed hypersensitivity

4. Which of the following disorders are known to be caused by autoantibodies (select all that apply)?

   a. Pernicious anemia
   b. Hay fever
   c. Insulin resistant diabetes mellitus
   d. Tuberculosis
   e. Myasthenia gravis

5. _____ means a person is prone to developing allergies because of hyperresponsiveness to sensitizing agents.

6. Which of the following are signs of allergic asthma (select all that apply)?

   a. Coughing after exercise
   b. Shortness of breath with exertion
   c. Chest tightness
   d. Rhinorrhea
   e. Coughing only in the morning

7. The diagnostic test that is considered the gold standard for establishing allergen-specific immunoglobulin E (IgE) antibodies is:

   a. Complete blood count (CBC)
   b. Purified-protein derivative (PPD)
   c. Antinuclear antibodies (ANA)
   d. Skin-prick test

8. Which of the following could interfere with the results of a skin-prick test?

   a. Steroids
   b. Nitroglycerin
   c. Antidepressants
   d. Antispasmodics

9. The cardinal principle in the therapeutic management of anaphylaxis is _____.

10. The medication most closely associated with anaphylactic shock and death is:

    a. Penicillin
    b. Coumadin
    c. Aspirin
    d. Augmentin

11. An allergy to _____ is the most common source of allergic rhinitis.

12. Which of the following is an example of allergic contact dermatitis?

    a. Wool rash
    b. Soap rash
    c. Latex allergy
    d. Synthetics rash

13. Which of the following are histamines used to treat urticaria (select all that apply)?

    a. Benadryl
    b. Aristocort
    c. Deltasone
    d. Atarax
    e. Vistaril

14. Which of the following could indicate a food allergy?

    a. If no immediate response, then not allergic to the food
    b. Gastric upset after eating spicy foods
    c. Lethargy after eating pasta
    d. Mouth itching while eating the food

15. A client exposed to poison ivy is at risk for developing:

    a. Hereditary angioedema
    b. Contact dermatitis
    c. Allergic rhinitis
    d. Serum sickness

Alterations in Integumentary Function

Assessment of Integumentary Function

1. List the two layers of the human skin.

   a. _____
   b. _____

2. Which of the following are epidermal appendages (select all that apply)?

   a. Carotenoids
   b. Eccrine glands
   c. Apocrine glands
   d. Hair follicles
   e. Merkel cells

3. The _____ tissue lies beneath the dermis and consists of fat cells.

4. The natural biochemical barrier of the skin is called the:

   a. Acid mantle
   b. Biodegradable shelf
   c. Macrophages
   d. Blood-brain barrier

5. The nurse realizes that the functions of the dermis include: (Select all that apply.)

   a. Preventing mechanical trauma
   b. Storing water
   c. Containing hair follicles
   d. Controlling temperature
   e. Housing sweat glands

6. _____ has natural antibacterial substances that retard growth of microorganisms.

7. Which of the following vitamins is synthesized through the skin through the use of UV light?

   a. Vitamin B_6
   b. Vitamin B_{12}
   c. Vitamin C
   d. Vitamin D

8. A client has a wound that extends deep into the dermis. The nurse realizes that the skin will repair this injury by:

   a. Replacing damaged cells with the same cell type
   b. Resurfacing the wound with epidermal cells
   c. Filling in the defect with dissimilar tissue
   d. Telangiectasias

9. _____ are flat brown spots seen on aged exposed skin.

10. List the three phases of wound healing.

    a. _____
    b. _____
    c. _____

11. Which of the following indicates a decrease in naturally produced skin lubricants?

    a. Ichthyosis
    b. Diaphoresis
    c. Turgor
    d. Anasarca

12. A greenish-blue drainage with a musty odor indicates a possible _____ infection.

13. Which of the following describes a confluent lesion?

    a. Individual, separate, and distinct
    b. Lesions merge and run together
    c. Lesions arranged in a circular pattern
    d. Lesions are clustered

14. Which of the following are considered secondary skin lesions (select all that apply)?

    a. Scars
    b. Nodules
    c. Wheals
    d. Pustules
    e. Scales

15. Which of the following lesions would be considered palpable?

    a. Macule
    b. Patch
    c. Vesicle
    d. Plaque

16. _____ micrographic surgery is a tissue-sparing method used to map tumors from frozen section.

17. A client is diagnosed with herpes zoster. Which of the following lesion configurations would the nurse most likely assess for this client?

    a. Eczematoid
    b. Iris
    c. Linear
    d. Dermatomal

Dermatological Dysfunction: Nursing Management

1. List the four methods used to debride necrotic tissue.

   a. _____
   b. _____
   c. _____
   d. _____

2. Which of the following medications is a suspension of an active ingredient and delivered under pressure?

   a. Aerosol
   b. Ointment
   c. Gel
   d. Powder

3. Which of the following will enhance the absorption of a topical medication?

   a. Rubbing it into the skin
   b. Opening the area to air
   c. Covering the area with an occlusive dressing
   d. Doing nothing

4. Vaseline gauze is an example of a _____ dressing.

5. Which of the following is responsible for the development of sunburn?

   a. Ultraviolet A
   b. Ultraviolet B
   c. Ultraviolet C
   d. Ultraviolet D

6. List the two groups into which contact dermatitis can be categorized.

   a. _____
   b. _____

7. Which of the following is a chronic fungal infection that appears as white patches on the skin?

   a. Tinea pedis
   b. Tinea cruris
   c. Tinea capitis
   d. Tinea versicolor

8. Which of the following are causes for age-related xerosis (select all that apply)?

   a. Water loss
   b. Human papilloma virus
   c. Venous insufficiency
   d. Decreased sebum production
   e. Vitamin C deficiency
   f. Unknown

9. List the most common types of skin cancer in the United States.

   a. _____
   b. _____

10. Which of the following should the nurse instruct a client who is prescribed a topical medication? (Select all that apply.)

    a. Apply ointment sparingly only to affected areas
    b. Apply medication after bathing or cleansing the area
    c. Apply directly to broken skin
    d. Avoid applying to face
    e. Cover area with moisture-retentive dressing

11. Which of the following is the treatment of choice for mild inflammatory acne?

    a. Topical antibiotics
    b. Sulfur
    c. Oral antibiotics
    d. Benzoyl peroxide

12. A potentially serious bacterial infection due to streptococcus or staphylococcus microorganisms that enter the skin through a wound or insect bite is considered _____.

13. Which of the following should be avoided in a client prone to developing pseudofolliculitis barbae?

    a. Close shaving
    b. Washing with soap
    c. Use of an electric razor
    d. Aftershave lotion

14. A client being treated for a carbuncle should expect which of the following as part of the treatment?

    a. Apply topical antibiotic
    b. Be prescribed oral antibiotics for 5 to 10 days
    c. Use cold compresses over the lesion
    d. Limit oral fluids

15. Which of the following instructions should a client diagnosed with head and body pediculosis receive regarding the treatment of the infestation?

    a. Apply the medication once
    b. Apply Kwell shampoo over the entire body
    c. Iron clothing along each seam
    d. Wash brushes and combs in cold soapy water

16. Which of the following will decrease inflammation associated with atopic dermatitis?

    a. Use of neutral pH soap
    b. Washing with a rough cloth
    c. Applying topical corticosteroid cream
    d. Taking antihistamines as prescribed

17. A client, diagnosed with mild rosacea, should be instructed regarding which of the following?

    a. Complete entire course of oral antibiotics
    b. Wash the face 5 times each day
    c. Use a firm washcloth when cleansing the face
    d. Avoid sunlight, alcohol, and spicy foods

CHAPTER 46

Burns: Nursing Management

1. List the four mechanisms of a burn injury.

    a. _____
    b. _____
    c. _____
    d. _____

2. Which of the following describes a third-degree burn?

    a. Superficial thickness
    b. Deep partial thickness
    c. Full thickness
    d. Split thickness

3. List the three zones of injury from a burn.

    a. _____
    b. _____
    c. _____

4. The first 24 to 48 hours after a burn injury is considered what phase of burn treatment?

    a. Emergent
    b. Acute
    c. Rehabilitation
    d. Hypermetabolism

5. The first intervention for a burn, regardless of the cause, is to _____ the burning process.

6. The pain medication of choice for a client with a burn injury is:

    a. Demerol
    b. Codeine
    c. Percodan
    d. Morphine sulfate

7. Which of the following is used to estimate the percentage of total body surface area burned?

    a. Rule of 12's
    b. Rule of 9's
    c. Rule of 7's
    d. Rule of 5's

8. Which of the following areas each equals 9 percent of a body surface area (select all that apply)?

    a. Neck
    b. Head
    c. Legs
    d. Posterior back and trunk
    e. Perineum
    f. Arms

9. A client who sustained a burn to the trunk and back is at risk for developing problems with:

    a. Breathing
    b. Recovery
    c. Movement
    d. Infection

10. A client with a burn injury has several firm, intact blisters. What should the nurse do with these blisters?

    a. Nothing
    b. Scratch them with sterile gauze
    c. Break them and apply a loose dressing
    d. Break them and debride the loose skin

11. A client with a circumferential burn might need a(n) _____, or linear surgical incisions to release the constriction from the burned tissue.

12. Which of the following are common complications seen in the acute period of burn management (select all that apply)?

    a. Stroke
    b. Infection
    c. Asthma
    d. Renal disease
    e. Heart failure

13. Which of the following terms defines the procedure in which layers of the burned area are shaved until the tissue begins to bleed?

    a. Xenograft
    b. Fascial technique
    c. Autograft
    d. Tangential excision

14. Which of the following would be beneficial for a client with a burn injury who is having difficulty adjusting to his or her post-burn appearance?

    a. Mood-altering medication
    b. Early ambulation
    c. Psychiatric consult
    d. Social services consult

15. The best indicator of adequate fluid resuscitation during the emergent phase of burn care is _____ _____.

16. Which of the following would prevent a client with a burn injury from being exposed to pseudomonas?

    a. Raw fruit consumption
    b. No live plants in the client's room
    c. Raw vegetable consumption
    d. No oral fluids

17. List four of the six most common behavioral reactions seen in a client with a burn injury.

    a. _____

    b. _____

    c. _____

    d. _____

18. The rehabilitative period of burn care begins:

    a. Two weeks after the date of the burn
    b. When the wound begins to itch
    c. When the client's weight stabilizes
    d. When the wound is closed

19. _____ is vital to the prevention of burn contractures.

20. Which of the following should be included in the instructions to a client with a burn who is prescribed an elastic pressure garment (select all that apply)?

    a. Wear for at least eight hours every day
    b. Wear the garment for six months to one year
    c. Remove the garment for one hour every day
    d. Use the garment until the first post-discharge health care provider's appointment
    e. Remove the garment during warm weather

Alterations in Gastrointestinal Function

CHAPTER 47

Assessment of Gastrointestinal Function

1. Saliva serves what purpose in the digestive process (select all that apply)?

   a. Allows a bolus of food to enter the esophagus
   b. Lubricates food
   c. Moves food to the stomach
   d. Dissolves food to enhance taste
   e. Mixes food

2. The gastric slow wave is _____ peristaltic waves per minute.

3. List the major digestive and absorptive areas of the gastrointestinal (GI) tract.

   a. _____
   b. _____
   c. _____

4. During the nutritional assessment, the nurse can also assess (select all that apply):

   a. Exercise pattern
   b. Bowel habits
   c. Abdominal pain
   d. Oral medications
   e. Activity pattern

5. Which of the following refers to difficulty in swallowing?

   a. Dyspepsia
   b. Aphasia
   c. Dysphagia
   d. Hemoptysis

6. The GI symptom that accounts for approximately 70 percent of all visits to a primary health care provider is:

   a. Pyrosis
   b. Odynophagia
   c. Dysphagia
   d. Dyspepsia

7. Which of the following should a client diagnosed with aerophagia be instructed to do (select all that apply)?

   a. Avoid alcohol
   b. Do not smoke
   c. Avoid carbonated beverages
   d. Increase milk consumption
   e. Eat slowly

8. Place in order the steps to follow when assessing the abdomen.

   a. Palpation
   b. Inspection
   c. Percussion
   d. Auscultation

9. A faint bluish color around the umbilicus, or _____ sign, can indicate intra-abdominal bleeding.

10. The two sounds heard when percussing the abdomen are (select all that apply):

    a. Tympany
    b. Resonance
    c. Hyperresonance
    d. Dull

11. A client diagnosed with acute appendicitis will have a positive:

    a. Blumberg's sign
    b. Cullen's sign
    c. Murphy's sign
    d. Fluid wave

12. The type of medication provided to conduct a colonoscopy is:

    a. General anesthesia
    b. Local anesthetic
    c. Conscious sedation
    d. Spinal anesthesia

13. Which of the following procedures is the aspiration of fluid from the abdominal cavity?

    a. Sigmoidoscopy
    b. Laparoscopy
    c. Lavage
    d. Paracentesis

14. Before inserting a nasogastric tube, the nurse should (select all that apply):

    a. Have the client sip water
    b. Check the gag reflex
    c. Anesthetize the client's throat
    d. Measure the length of the tube to be inserted
    e. Assess for a patent nostril

15. The best way to keep a feeding tube patent is to:

    a. Do nothing
    b. Flush it with water
    c. Provide an air bolus after using
    d. Flush with normal saline

CHAPTER 48

Nutrition, Malnutrition, and Obesity: Nursing Management

1. List the three leading causes of preventable death.

   a. _____
   b. _____
   c. _____

2. The process of carbohydrate digestion begins in the:

   a. Esophagus
   b. Stomach
   c. Mouth
   d. Duodenum

3. How many minutes of exercise per day are needed to attain active lifestyle?

   a. 10
   b. 15
   c. 30
   d. 60

4. When an individual is in energy balance:

   a. Body weight stays the same
   b. Weight decreases
   c. Weight increases
   d. Thirst increases

5. The liver enzymes _____ and _____ participate in drug metabolism.

6. A client receiving Coumadin should be instructed to avoid which of the following foods (select all that apply)?

   a. Chicken
   b. Liver
   c. Spinach
   d. Bananas
   e. Apples
   f. Cherries

7. The term that refers to providing nutrition through a feeding tube is:

   a. Parenteral
   b. Supplemental
   c. Enteral
   d. Oral

8. Which of the following are appropriate interventions for a client receiving tube feeding (select all that apply)?

   a. Keep head of bed flat during the feeding
   b. Elevate the head of bed 30 degrees for 1 hour after the feeding
   c. Flush the tube with water before and after the feeding
   d. Check the gag reflex before each feeding
   e. Assess vital signs before each feeding

9. Malnutrition in hospitalized clients is usually caused by:

   a. Undernutrition
   b. Overnutrition
   c. Enzyme deficiency
   d. Fluid deficit

10. _____, or long-term undernutrition, is characterized by tissue wasting, dehydration, and weight loss.

11. Which diagnostic test will best identify a short-term change in nutritional status?

    a. Serum transferrin
    b. Prealbumin
    c. Retinol binding protein
    d. Albumin

12. Obesity is defined as a body mass index of:

    a. Less than 18.5
    b. 18.5 to 25
    c. 25 to 29.9
    d. Greater than 30

13. An obese client with a body mass index of 33 should decrease caloric intake by 300 to 500 calories per day to achieve what percentage of weight loss in 6 months?

    a. 10 percent
    b. 20 percent
    c. 30 percent
    d. 40 percent

14. The most common type of bariatric surgery performed in the United States is:

    a. Adjustable banding
    b. Roux-en-Y
    c. Vertical banding
    d. Esophageal stapling

15. A bariatric surgery client may experience _____ _____ if high-carbohydrate foods are consumed.

16. A diet that is rich in fruits, vegetables, nuts, and seeds but low in poultry, dairy, fish, and meat is often called the:

    a. Atkins' diet
    b. South Beach diet
    c. Zone diet
    d. Mediterranean diet

Upper Gastrointestinal Tract Dysfunction: Nursing Management

1. Unusually loud hyperactive bowel tones are considered _____.

2. Which of the following would be considered outcome criteria for the nursing diagnosis of *Imbalanced nutrition: Less than body requirements* during the evaluation of care for a client diagnosed with stomach cancer?

   a. Verbalization of adequate pain relief
   b. Absence of purulent drainage from wounds
   c. Client weight is within 10 percent of ideal body weight
   d. Demonstrate positive coping mechanisms

3. Which of the following are true of burning mouth syndrome (select all that apply)?

   a. Relieved by eating and drinking
   b. Will stop within 10 to 14 days
   c. Caused by a systemic disease
   d. Is a type of neuropathy
   e. Produces visible red patches on the tongue

4. The gold standard for evaluating dysphagia is _____, or modified barium swallow.

5. Which of the following is indicated for a client with a risk for aspiration or regurgitation?

   a. Thick foods
   b. Mechanical soft diet
   c. Pureed diet
   d. No eating at bedtime

6. List the three types of swallowing therapy.

   a. _____
   b. _____
   c. _____

7. A client diagnosed with Barrett's esophagus might experience a sensation of saliva filling the mouth. This is also called:

   a. Brash water
   b. Dyspepsia
   c. Aphagia
   d. Pyrosis

8. Which of the following medications are proton pump inhibitors (select all that apply)?

   a. Pepcid
   b. Tagamet
   c. Prilosec
   d. Zantac
   e. Prevacid

9. List the two primary types of hiatal hernia.

   a. _____
   b. _____

10. Which of the following major medication classifications are associated with dyspepsia (select all that apply)?

    a. Nonsteroidal anti-inflammatory drugs (NSAIDs)
    b. Antibiotics
    c. Aspirin
    d. Angiotensin-converting enzyme (ACE) inhibitors
    e. Calcium channel blockers

11. The most common cause linked to peptic ulcer dyspepsia is:

    a. Hiatal hernia
    b. *Helicobacter pylori*
    c. Use of nitroglycerin
    d. Lactose intolerance

12. There are _____ types of gastric ulcers.

13. The major presenting symptom of peptic ulcer disease is:

    a. Nausea
    b. Vomiting
    c. Diarrhea
    d. Pain

14. A client diagnosed with non–*H. pylori* peptic ulcer disease must take NSAIDs. Which of the following can this client be prescribed to heal the stomach ulcers?

    a. Antacids
    b. Proton pump inhibitors
    c. Hydrogen ion receptor agonists
    d. Antibiotics

15. Which of the following foods may protect against the development of stomach cancer (select all that apply)?

    a. Pickled herring
    b. Smoked sausage
    c. Fresh oranges
    d. Frozen strawberries
    e. Salted cod

Lower Gastrointestinal Tract Dysfunction: Nursing Management

1. Which of the following is a source of natural vitamin B_{12}?

   a. Milk
   b. Green vegetables
   c. Chicken
   d. Meat

2. A client diagnosed with steatorrhea has a dysfunction in the metabolism of:

   a. Fat
   b. Protein
   c. Carbohydrates
   d. Folic acid

3. What causes mal-assimilation disorders?

   a. Mal _____
   b. Mal _____

4. Which of the following are seen in a client diagnosed with a mal-assimilation disorder (select all that apply)?

   a. Increased libido
   b. Weight loss
   c. Bleeding gums
   d. Negative Babinski reflex
   e. Fatigue
   f. Dandruff

5. The most commonly missed diagnoses of an acute abdomen are _____ and _____.

6. List the three major pathological processes of acute abdomen.

   a. _____
   b. _____
   c. _____

7. The symptom triad of generalized abdominal pain, board-like rigidity, and rebound tenderness indicates:

    a. Appendicitis
    b. Peritonitis
    c. Peptic ulcer disease
    d. Abdominal hernia

8. Which of the following are primary, acute inflammatory disorders of the lower gastrointestinal (GI) tract? (Select all that apply.)

    a. Diverticulitis
    b. Ruptured visus
    c. Kidney stones
    d. Appendicitis
    e. Abdominal aortic aneurysm

9. A distressing but ineffectual urge to evacuate the rectum is called _____.

10. The development of diverticular disease is linked to: (Select all that apply.)

    a. Vegetable consumption
    b. Low-fiber diet
    c. Diet high in refined foods
    d. Raw fish consumption
    e. Sedentary lifestyle

11. Which of the following should be suspected if bowel sounds cannot be auscultated?

    a. Ileus
    b. Diverticulitis
    c. Appendicitis
    d. Peptic ulcer disease

12. The most common cause of small bowel obstruction is:

    a. Constipation
    b. Dehydration
    c. Postoperative abdominal adhesions
    d. Laxative abuse

13. How often should a colonoscopy to screen for colon rectal cancer be conducted?

    a. Every year after age 50
    b. Every 3 years after age 50
    c. Every 5 years after age 50
    d. Every 10 years after age 50

14. A bulging stoma would indicate:

    a. Nothing
    b. A developing hernia
    c. An obstruction
    d. A fecal impaction

15. Which of the following medications have been effective when treating irritable bowel syndrome (select all that apply)?

    a. Angiotensin-converting enzyme (ACE) inhibitors
    b. Nicotinic acid
    c. Bulk-forming laxatives
    d. Antidepressants
    e. Antiemetics
    f. Peppermint

16. Name two chronic inflammatory bowel disorders.

    a. _____

    b. _____

17. Which of the following is the first medication used to treat Crohn's disease?

    a. Aminosalicylates
    b. Corticosteroids
    c. Immunomodulatory agents
    d. Monoclonal antibodies

Hepatic, Biliary Tract, and Pancreatic Dysfunction: Nursing Management

1. The functional unit of the liver is the _____.

2. Which of the following serum blood tests is the most useful to diagnose the cause of jaundice?

   a. Prothrombin time
   b. Ammonia
   c. Amylase
   d. Alkaline phosphatase

3. List the three stages of hepatitis.

   a. _____
   b. _____
   c. _____

4. The type of hepatitis that health care workers are most prone to contracting is:

   a. A
   b. B
   c. C
   d. E

5. The most common nonviral source of inflammatory hepatitis is:

   a. Alcohol
   b. Nonsteroidal anti-inflammatory drugs (NSAIDs)
   c. Antibiotics
   d. Allergies

6. The common causes of cirrhosis are (select all that apply):

   a. Copper toxicity
   b. Protein malabsorption
   c. Hepatitis infections
   d. Drug-induced
   e. Hemochromatosis
   f. Alcohol

7. The term used to describe liver sweat is _____.

8. Medications used to treat refractory ascites include (select all that apply):

    a. Betapace
    b. Spironolactone
    c. Inderal
    d. Dilantin
    e. Furosemide

9. Which of the following is used to treat portal-systemic encephalopathy?

    a. Mannitol
    b. Spironolactone
    c. Furosemide
    d. Lactulose

10. The most common finding of a fatty liver is _____.

11. Most people with liver trauma are treated:

    a. Medically, without surgery
    b. With stent placement
    c. With a liver resection
    d. With a transcatheter embolization

12. Which of the following are clinical manifestations of liver cancer (select all that apply)?

    a. Right upper quadrant pain
    b. Right shoulder pain
    c. Positive Murphy's sign
    d. Jaundice
    e. Weight loss

13. List the two types of liver transplantation.

    a. _____
    b. _____

14. A symptom of liver transplantation rejection is:

    a. Diarrhea
    b. Jaundice
    c. Low blood sugar
    d. Thirst

15. The most useful test to diagnose cholelithiasis is:

    a. Abdominal X-ray
    b. Liver spleen scan
    c. Barium swallow
    d. Ultrasound

16. Serum tests used to diagnose acute pancreatitis include (select all that apply):

    a. Serum lipase
    b. Bilirubin
    c. Prothrombin time
    d. Hematocrit
    e. Serum amylase

Alterations in Renal Function

Assessment of Renal Function

1. List the four anatomical structures of the renal system.

   a. _____

   b. _____

   c. _____

   d. _____

2. The kidneys are located in the _____ space.

3. The renal arteries are branches from:

   a. The inferior vena cava
   b. The superior vena cava
   c. The pulmonary veins
   d. The aorta

4. The landmark used to locate kidney position during a physical examination is called:

   a. Erb's point
   b. Costovertebral angle
   c. Angle of Louis
   d. None of the above

5. Which of the following are functions of the kidney (select all that apply)?

   a. Blood pressure regulation
   b. Metabolize vitamin C
   c. Create red blood cells
   d. Maintain fluid balance
   e. Store chemicals

6. The functioning unit of the kidney is the _____.

7. Which of the following do healthy glomerular capillaries prevent the passage of into the urine (select all that apply)?

   a. Carbohydrates
   b. Blood cells
   c. Protein
   d. Sodium
   e. Water

8. Which of the following is an age-related change seen in the renal system?

    a. Incontinence because of poor muscle tone
    b. Increased thirst
    c. Low urine output
    d. Renal calculi

9. Which of the following are considered nephrotoxic (select all that apply)?

    a. Amoxicillin
    b. Contrast medium
    c. NSAIDs
    d. Penicillin
    e. Gentamycin

10. A weight gain of 1 kg could indicate the retention of _____ liter(s) of fluid.

11. A bacterial count greater than 100,000 in a urine culture indicates:

    a. Nothing
    b. A contaminated specimen
    c. An infection
    d. A kidney stone

12. Which of the following serum tests is more reliable than the blood urea nitrogen (BUN) for indicating renal dysfunction?

    a. Serum creatinine
    b. Serum sodium
    c. Serum potassium
    d. Serum phosphorous

13. List the two ways to assess postvoid residual urine.

    a. _____
    b. _____

14. Which of the following can be given to a client prescribed a fluid-restriction, who is scheduled for a diagnostic test with a nephrotoxic contrast agent?

    a. Aspirin
    b. Normal saline
    c. Heparin
    d. Sodium bicarbonate

15. Painful urination, or _____, might occur after a cystoscopy and should be reported to the health care provider.

CHAPTER 53

Urinary Dysfunction: Nursing Management

1. One way to label urinary tract infections (UTIs) is according to the region. Name the general region terms.

   a. _____
   b. _____

2. Which of the following can cause a UTI? (Select all that apply.)

   a. *Escherichia coli*
   b. Oral birth control bills
   c. Low fluid intake
   d. Urinary tract obstruction
   e. Incomplete bladder emptying

3. Which of the following are clinical manifestations of a lower UTI? (Select all that apply.)

   a. Fever over 101° F (38.3° C)
   b. Dysuria
   c. Foul-smelling urine
   d. Nausea
   e. Vomiting

4. A client prescribed Bactrim for a UTI should be instructed to:

   a. Avoid antacids
   b. Take with food
   c. Take with milk
   d. Drink large amounts of fluid

5. _____, or urination at night, is one symptom of interstitial cystitis.

6. List the two groups of interstitial cystitis.

   a. _____
   b. _____

7. The first test often used to check for interstitial cystitis is:

   a. Urine specimen
   b. Urine culture
   c. Bladder scan
   d. Cystoscopy

8. If left untreated, pyelonephritis can potentially lead to:

   a. Renal failure
   b. Kidney stones
   c. Bladder cancer
   d. Interstitial cystitis

9. Which of the following are manifestations of glomerulonephritis? (Select all that apply.)

   a. Dark, cola-colored urine
   b. Thirst
   c. Periorbital edema in the morning
   d. Hypertension
   e. Leg cramps

10. List the three major symptoms seen in nephrotic syndrome.

    a. _____
    b. _____
    c. _____

11. The primary goal of care for a client diagnosed with nephrotic syndrome is to:

    a. Adjust acid-base balance
    b. Preserve renal function
    c. Reduce fluid overload
    d. Improve circulation

12. A client diagnosed with sterile pyuria and hematuria should be evaluated for:

    a. Nephrotic syndrome
    b. Interstitial cystitis
    c. Renal tuberculosis
    d. UTI

13. _____ are urinary tract stones, whereas _____ are stones in the kidney.

14. The causes of staghorn calculi are: (Select all that apply.)

    a. Calcium
    b. Magnesium
    c. Uric acid
    d. Phosphate
    e. Ammonium

15. The first priority of care for a client diagnosed with a renal stone is:

    a. Pain control
    b. Nutritional intake
    c. Bedrest
    d. Blood pressure control

16. Which of the following is considered the cardinal sign of renal trauma?

    a. Flank pain
    b. Renal colic
    c. Pyuria
    d. Hematuria

17. List the three primary renal vascular disorders.

    a. _____
    b. _____
    c. _____

18. The first step in treating a client diagnosed with renal cancer is:

    a. Full or partial kidney removal
    b. Radiation
    c. Chemotherapy
    d. Immunotherapy

19. A client diagnosed with bladder cancer who needs a cystectomy will likely need:

    a. Rehabilitation
    b. A urinary system diversion
    c. Long-term antibiotic therapy
    d. Heparinization

20. List the four types of stress incontinence.

    a. _____
    b. _____
    c. _____
    d. _____

CHAPTER 54

Renal Dysfunction: Nursing Management

1. An infection of the upper urinary tract, or _____, is commonly caused by urinary retention.

2. To diagnose pyelonephritis in a client who is experiencing renal compromise, the diagnostic tool of choice is:

    a. Ultrasound
    b. Computed tomography (CT) scan
    c. Intravenous pyelogram (IVP)
    d. Magnetic resonance imaging (MRI)

3. Nursing care to prevent the onset of urinary tract infections in clients diagnosed with pyelonephritis include: (Select all that apply.)

    a. Urinary catheters for incontinent clients
    b. Hand washing
    c. Restricting fluids
    d. Strict aseptic technique with urinary catheter insertion
    e. Enforcing bedrest

4. Which of the following is a genetically inherited kidney disease?

    a. Pyelonephritis
    b. Interstitial cystitis
    c. Kidney stones
    d. Polycystic kidney disease

5. Because cardiovascular complications are the primary cause of death in clients diagnosed with polycystic kidney disease, treatment is often aimed at:

    a. Blood pressure control
    b. Infection control
    c. Nutritional status
    d. Gastrointestinal (GI) functioning

6. List the three genetic forms of Alport syndrome.

    a. _____
    b. _____
    c. _____

7. The disease Wegener granulomatosis often presents as:

   a. Abdominal pain
   b. Diarrhea
   c. A respiratory illness
   d. Nothing

8. Anti-glomerular basement membrane disease can be exacerbated by exposure to:

   a. Milk
   b. Cigarette smoke
   c. Red meat
   d. Amoxicillin

9. A client with multiple crush injuries is prone to developing:

   a. Rhabdomyolysis
   b. Interstitial cystitis
   c. Renal calculi
   d. Urinary retention

10. List the classifications of acute renal failure.

    a. _____
    b. _____
    c. _____

11. Which of the following is evidence of acute renal failure? (Select all that apply.)

    a. Elevated blood urea nitrogen (BUN)
    b. Low uric acid level
    c. Elevated calcium level
    d. Oliguria
    e. Drop in red blood cells

12. Which of the following are intrarenal causes of acute renal failure? (Select all that apply.)

    a. Vitamin K deficiency
    b. Nonsteroidal anti-inflammatory drugs (NSAIDs)
    c. Angiotensin-converting enzyme (ACE) inhibitors
    d. Weight reduction diets
    e. Contrast dye

13. There are _____ stages of chronic kidney disease based on glomerular filtration rates.

14. A buildup of nitrogenous waste products on the skin is called:

    a. Necrosis
    b. Eschar
    c. Azotemia
    d. Keloid

15. The three treatment options available to a client diagnosed with chronic kidney failure are:

    a. _____
    b. _____
    c. _____

16. To confirm the patency of an arteriovenous fistula, the nurse should:

    a. Measure the client's blood pressure above the fistula
    b. Perform venipuncture through the fistula
    c. Place an intravenous (IV) access device above the level of the fistula
    d. Palpate for a thrill

17. A client receiving peritoneal dialysis is experiencing cloudy effluent. This means:

    a. Nothing
    b. More dialysate must be instilled.
    c. Peritonitis could be developing.
    d. The kidneys are responding to the treatment.

Alterations in Endocrine Function

Assessment of Endocrine Function

1. _____ are chemical messengers produced and secreted by endocrine cells.

2. The most common type of feedback system found within the endocrine system is:

   a. Positive
   b. Potentiating
   c. Negative
   d. Propagating

3. Which of the following are considered endocrine glands? (Select all that apply.)

   a. Thyroid
   b. Sweat
   c. Lacrimal
   d. Pituitary
   e. Adrenals

4. Tissues or organs in the body that are affected by specific hormones are the:

   a. Exocrine glands
   b. Target tissues
   c. End organs
   d. Endocrine glands

5. The function of the thyroid hormones triiodothyronine (T3) and thyroxine (T4) is to:

   a. Decrease blood glucose level
   b. Raise blood glucose level
   c. Raise metabolic rate
   d. Decrease blood calcium level

6. In a positive feedback mechanism, when the level of one hormone increases, another hormone will:

   a. Stay the same
   b. Decrease
   c. Increase
   d. Activate white blood cell formation

7. The major regulating organ of the body is the _____.

8. Which of the following is considered the master gland?

   a. Pituitary
   b. Hypothalamus
   c. Pancreas
   d. Thyroid

9. The hormones produced in the posterior pituitary gland are: (Select all that apply.)

   a. Growth hormones
   b. Thyroid stimulating hormones (TSHs)
   c. Luteinizing hormones
   d. Oxytocin
   e. Antidiuretic hormones (ADHs)

10. Of the two thyroid hormones, the most powerful is T3 or _____.

11. The hormone that increases the blood glucose level is:

    a. Cortisol
    b. Calcitonin
    c. Aldosterone
    d. Parathyroid

12. List the four types of cells within the islets of Langerhans.

    a. _____
    b. _____
    c. _____
    d. _____

13. The hormone produced by the beta cells within the pancreas is:

    a. ADH
    b. Insulin
    c. Aldosterone
    d. Cortisol

14. As a person ages, the thyroid gland becomes smaller causing a(n):

    a. Increase in metabolic rate
    b. Decrease in ADH absorption
    c. Increase in calcium storage
    d. Decrease in metabolic rate

15. Eye bulging, or _____, is associated with Grave's disease.

Endocrine Dysfunction: Nursing Management

1. A client experiencing visual changes should have which of the following glands evaluated for enlargement?

   a. Pituitary
   b. Hypothalamus
   c. Thyroid
   d. Parathyroid

2. The condition in adults caused by hypersecretion of growth hormone is_____.

3. A client diagnosed with acromegaly is prone to developing:

   a. Thyroid cancer
   b. Diabetes
   c. Renal failure
   d. Spontaneous fractures

4. Cushing's disease is caused by:

   a. Excessive adrenocorticotropin hormone
   b. Excessive growth hormone
   c. Decreased antidiuretic hormone (ADH)
   d. Elevated thyroxine (T4)

5. Which of the following are manifestations of Cushing's disease (select all that apply)?

   a. Scoliosis
   b. Thin extremities
   c. Buffalo hump
   d. Pale complexion
   e. Hirsutism

6. The treatment of choice for Cushing's disease is:

   a. Medication therapy
   b. Bilateral adrenalectomy
   c. Transsphenoidal resection
   d. Radiation therapy

7. A client recovering from an oral transsphenoidal hypophysectomy has clear nasal drainage. This drainage would indicate a cerebral spinal fluid leak if: (Select all that apply.)

   a. The client starts to seize.
   b. The drainage tests positive for glucose.
   c. The drainage creates a halo ring on a gauze pad.
   d. The drainage tests negative for glucose.
   e. The drainage creates a star pattern on a gauze pad.

8. Primary adrenal insufficiency, or _____, disease is rare.

9. Which of the following is a hallmark clinical manifestation of primary Addison's disease?

   a. Pallor
   b. Cyanosis
   c. Erythema
   d. Hyperpigmentation

10. Physical manifestations of hyperaldosteronism include:

    a. Hypotension
    b. Nothing
    c. Reduced urine output
    d. Craving licorice

11. A rare disorder that causes severe hypertension caused by an adrenal gland tumor is a
    (n) _____.

12. The most common and sensitive test for pheochromocytoma is:

    a. Renal ultrasound
    b. Serum free metanephrine level
    c. Magnetic resonance imaging (MRI)
    d. Computed tomography (CT) scan

13. List five of the nine causes of hypopituitarism.

    a. _____
    b. _____
    c. _____
    d. _____
    e. _____

14. The primary symptoms of diabetes insipidus are (select all that apply):

    a. Thirst for ice water
    b. Polyphagia
    c. Nausea
    d. Hair loss
    e. Polyuria up to 20 liters per day

15. The best diagnostic test to indicate thyroid function is:

    a. Serum thyroxine (T4)
    b. Serum triiodothyronine (T3)
    c. Thyroid-stimulating hormone (TSH) level
    d. Thyroid antibodies

16. Which of the following are indicated for a client experiencing thyroid storm (select all that apply)?

    a. Do not provide with aspirin
    b. Keep on nothing by mouth (NPO) status
    c. Provide acetaminophen
    d. Provide intravenous (IV) fluids
    e. Provide ice water

17. A client with an elevated T4 level might be prescribed:

    a. Propyl-Thyracil
    b. Atenolol
    c. Potassium iodide
    d. PIMA

18. If a client has not responded to antithyroid therapy for hyperthyroidism, the next treatment of choice is:

    a. Thyroid radiation
    b. Chemotherapy
    c. Radioiodine therapy
    d. Thyroidectomy

19. Which of the following are manifestations of hypothyroidism? (Select all that apply.)

    a. Oily skin
    b. Hoarseness
    c. Shallow respirations
    d. Tachycardia
    e. Dry skin

20. A hallmark sign of primary hyperparathyroidism is an elevated serum _____ level.

CHAPTER 57

Diabetes Mellitus: Nursing Management

1. List the most common types of diabetes.

    a. _____
    b. _____
    c. _____

2. Which cells of the pancreas produce glucagon?

    a. Alpha
    b. Beta
    c. Delta
    d. F

3. Manifestations of Metabolic Syndrome include (select all that apply):

    a. Elevated triglycerides
    b. Weight loss
    c. Muscle wasting
    d. Elevated low-density lipoproteins (LDLs)
    e. Low high-density lipoproteins (HDLs)

4. List the three Ps of diabetes.

    a. _____
    b. _____
    c. _____

5. If a client has a random plasma glucose level greater than 200 mg/dL, what should be done?

    a. Nothing
    b. Begin treatment for diabetes
    c. Draw a blood sample for a hemoglobin A1c level
    d. Assess for use of an insulin pump

6. Which of the following is a reason NPH insulin may appear cloudy?

    a. It has crossed the expiry date.
    b. It has additives.
    c. It has been contaminated with regular insulin.
    d. It has been refrigerated.

7. If a client receives a dose of Lispro insulin, what must be done next?

   a. Exercise
   b. Eat within one hour
   c. Continue normal activities of daily living
   d. Eat within 15 minutes

8. Place the following anatomical sites in order of the speed of absorption of insulin:

   a. Thighs
   b. Abdomen
   c. Buttocks
   d. Arms

9. Which of the following should the nurse instruct a client diagnosed with type 2 diabetes mellitus regarding medication therapy?

   a. The medication is in addition to diet and exercise
   b. The medication will cure the diabetes
   c. Insulin is not needed to treat type 2 diabetes mellitus
   d. Limit excess activity and increase rest throughout the day

10. Alcohol intake can lead to _____, so the client should eat while drinking.

11. _____ is a lumpy area on the skin caused by repeated insulin injections.

12. The treatment of choice for a client experiencing the Symogi effect is to:

    a. Reduce insulin dose
    b. Only use regular insulin
    c. Increase insulin dose
    d. Only use Lispro

13. In diabetic ketoacidosis (DKA), the production of ketones can cause the client to develop:

    a. Respiratory acidosis
    b. Respiratory alkalosis
    c. Metabolic acidosis
    d. Metabolic alkalosis

14. In DKA, the client will exhibit an acetone, or _____, breath odor.

15. A client diagnosed with type 2 diabetes is admitted to the hospital with a blood glucose of 560 mg/dL without urine ketones. This patient is demonstrating symptoms of:

    a. DKA
    b. Acute renal failure
    c. Hyperosmolar hyperglycemic nonketotic syndrome (HHNS)
    d. Hypoglycemia

16. A client who is unable to detect his or her own low blood sugar might be experiencing _____ _____.

17. In which of the following will microvascular complications of diabetes be manifested (select all that apply)?

    a. Eyes
    b. Blood vessels
    c. Heart
    d. Skin
    e. Kidneys

18. List the two most common types of diabetic neuropathies.

    a. _____

    b. _____

19. The most common cause of hospitalization for the client diagnosed with diabetes is:

    a. Heart attack
    b. Pneumonia
    c. Wounds on the feet
    d. Urinary tract infection

Alterations in Musculoskeletal Function

CHAPTER 58

Assessment of Musculoskeletal Function

1. List the four types of bones in the body.

   a. _____
   b. _____
   c. _____
   d. _____

2. The type of mature bone that is hard and forms the protective exterior portion of all bones is:

   a. Cancellous
   b. Cortical
   c. Trabecular
   d. Spongy

3. Which of the following is the bone cell responsible for building bone?

   a. Osteoclasts
   b. Osteocytes
   c. Cytokines
   d. Osteoblasts

4. Of the five physiological processes of bone, which describes bone turnover at the microscopic level?

   a. Remodeling
   b. Repair
   c. Growth
   d. Modeling

5. After a bone fracture, the stage of ossification can take what length of time to complete?

   a. 24 to 48 hours
   b. 2 to 3 weeks
   c. 3 to 4 months
   d. Years

6. If not treated, _____ may result in osteoporosis.

7. Which of the following are synovial fluid-filled sacs located near joints?

   a. Myosin
   b. Bursae
   c. Tendons
   d. Ligaments

8. List the three classifications of joints.

   a. _____
   b. _____
   c. _____

9. Of the following, choose the items needed to conduct a musculoskeletal assessment (select all that apply):

   a. Flashlight
   b. Stethoscope
   c. Goniometer
   d. Penlight
   e. Tape measure

10. Which of the following are vital focus areas when completing an adult orthopedic musculoskeletal health history (select all that apply)?

    a. Range of motion
    b. Pain
    c. Gait
    d. Deformity
    e. Strength

11. A _____ _____ is a fracture in which the bones have gone out of natural alignment.

12. A client is able to perform range of motion with gravity but without added resistance. This client's muscle strength is graded as:

    a. 0
    b. 1
    c. 2
    d. 3

13. List the two phases of gait.

    a. _____
    b. _____

14. Which of the following laboratory tests is used to evaluate inflammation in a client experiencing degenerative arthritis?

    a. Calcium
    b. Aldolase
    c. Erythrocyte sedimentation rate (ESR)
    d. Uric acid

15. Which of the following tests is used to relieve pain in a joint cavity?

    a. Joint aspirate
    b. Bone scan
    c. Nerve conduction studies
    d. Angiogram

16. The test used to assist in the early diagnosis of osteoporosis is the _____ _____ scan.

Musculoskeletal Dysfunction: Nursing Management

1. The most common form of joint disease is _____, or degenerative joint disease.

2. Which of the following are manifestations of osteoarthritis (select all that apply)?

   a. Joint pain
   b. Pain at rest
   c. Pain at night
   d. Crepitus
   e. Effects the wrists

3. Which of the following would be indicated for a client who is not receiving pain control with acetaminophen for osteoarthritis?

   a. Aspirin
   b. Nonsteroidal anti-inflammatory drugs (NSAIDs)
   c. Opioids
   d. Tramadol

4. Which of the following nutritional supplements has been beneficial to clients diagnosed with osteoarthritis (select all that apply)?

   a. Hypericum
   b. Vitamin C
   c. Vitamin D
   d. St. John's wort
   e. Calcium

5. Which of the following is a cause of primary gout?

   a. Obesity
   b. Lead toxicity
   c. Excessive purine synthesis
   d. Diuretics

6. List the four categories of medications to treat gout.

   a. _____
   b. _____
   c. _____
   d. _____

7. A client diagnosed with Lyme disease will have a circular bullseye rash, or _____ _____.

8. Which of the following should be included when instructing a client about Lyme disease? (Select all that apply.)

   a. Complete the entire course of antibiotics.
   b. Arthritis pain is seen in the early stage of the disease.
   c. NSAIDs are the treatment of choice.
   d. Use insect repellent with diethyltoluamide (DEET).
   e. There is no known cure.

9. The spinal X-ray of a client diagnosed with advancing ankylosing spondylitis will show:

   a. Bone spurs
   b. Bamboo spine
   c. Narrowing of the vertebral column
   d. Nothing

10. In which of the following arthritic conditions is a "sausage toe" a classic symptom?

    a. Ankylosing spondylitis
    b. Reactive arthritis
    c. Psoriatic arthritis
    d. Reiter's syndrome

11. List the three hallmark tests used to confirm dermatomyositis and polymyositis.

    a. _____
    b. _____
    c. _____

12. To diagnose fibromyalgia, how many common tender points need to test positive?

    a. 5
    b. 8
    c. 11
    d. 18

13. Because osteoporosis is often considered a silent disease, the first indication of a problem might be:

    a. A fracture
    b. A blood clot
    c. A heart attack
    d. A hiatal hernia

14. Which of the following are included in the treatment of osteoporosis? (Select all that apply.)

    a. Use of bisphosphonates
    b. Reduce red meat consumption
    c. Use of steroids
    d. Follow a low purine diet
    e. Weight-bearing exercises

15. Which of the following tests are used to diagnose Paget's disease? (Select all that apply.)

    a. Magnetic resonance imaging (MRI)
    b. Serum alkaline phosphatase
    c. Bone scan
    d. X-ray
    e. Computed tomography (CT) scan

16. _____, or a bone infection, is considered chronic if it lasts longer than _____ months.

17. Which of the following is a soft tissue tumor that is commonly located in and around the knee joint?

    a. Tendosynovial sarcoma
    b. Liposarcoma
    c. Fibrosarcoma
    d. Ewing's sarcoma

18. The definitive diagnostic test for a sarcoma is a(n):

    a. MRI
    b. Biopsy
    c. CT scan
    d. X-ray

19. A test used to assess for scoliosis is the Adam's _____ test.

CHAPTER 60

Musculoskeletal Trauma: Nursing Management

1. The initial treatment of sports-related injuries includes RICE, which stands for what?

   a. R = _____
   b. I = _____
   c. C = _____
   d. E = _____

2. Which of the following are factors associated with overuse syndrome? (Select all that apply.)

   a. Obesity
   b. Repetitive tasks
   c. Exposure to cold
   d. Vitamin C deficiency
   e. Boredom

3. The goals of treatment for a rotator cuff tear are (select all that apply):

   a. Rest
   b. Increase joint mobility with range of motion exercises
   c. Low-fat diet to lower lipid levels
   d. Reduce inflammation with steroids
   e. Immobilization

4. The most common cause of compression neuropathy of the upper extremity is:

   a. Carpal tunnel syndrome
   b. Patellar tendinopathy
   c. Anterior cruciate ligament tear
   d. Lateral epicondylitis

5. List the two classic tests used to help diagnose carpal tunnel syndrome.

   a. _____
   b. _____

6. Which of the following are indicated for patellar tendinopathy? (Select all that apply.)

   a. Immobilize the joint
   b. Avoid jumping
   c. Avoid squatting
   d. Steroid injections
   e. Nothing

7. The main complication of a knee ligament injury is:

   a. Ongoing instability
   b. Paralysis
   c. Deep vein thrombosis
   d. Bleeding

8. The most common type of ankle sprain is a(n):

   a. Medial
   b. Lateral
   c. Dorsal
   d. Extension

9. Tests used to diagnose the stability of an ankle joint after injury include: (Select all that apply.)

   a. Magnetic resonance imaging (MRI)
   b. Inversion stress test
   c. Computed tomography (CT) scan
   d. Romberg's test
   e. Drawer test

10. The strongest tendon in the body is the _____ tendon.

11. Injury to the Achilles tendon is seen most frequently in:

    a. Football
    b. Soccer
    c. Tennis
    d. Polo

12. The test used to help diagnose a ruptured Achilles tendon is the:

    a. Inversion stress test
    b. Drawer test
    c. CT scan
    d. Thompson test

13. If left untreated, which of the following can occur in a client experiencing plantar fasciitis?

    a. Loss of function
    b. Paralysis
    c. Chronic pain
    d. Nothing

14. Stress fractures are most commonly seen in:

    a. Basketball
    b. Track and field sports
    c. Tennis
    d. Football

15. Fractures can be classified in what two ways?

    a. _____
    b. _____

16. The use of percutaneous pins or wires to stabilize a fracture is called:

    a. Open reduction
    b. Closed reduction
    c. External fixation
    d. Internal fixation

17. Which of the following should be included when instructing a client with a cast? (Select all that apply.)

    a. Do not scratch under the cast.
    b. Inspect the cast daily.
    c. Foul odors from the cast are expected.
    d. Avoid elevating the casted limb.
    e. Tightness is normal.

18. If a client diagnosed with a femoral neck hip fracture goes without treatment, which of the following can develop?

    a. Avascular necrosis
    b. Infection
    c. Bleeding
    d. Deep vein thrombosis

19. Which of the following are classic symptoms of fat emboli? (Select all that apply.)

    a. Petechiae
    b. Increased blood pressure
    c. Hypoxemia
    d. Mental status changes
    e. Joint pain

20. A client recovering from a limb amputation complains of pain in the ankle of the amputated limb. This type of pain is:

    a. Residual limb
    b. Phantom limb
    c. Chronic limb
    d. Neuropathic limb

Alterations in Reproductive Function

CHAPTER 61

Assessment of Reproductive Function

1. List the primary functions of the male reproductive system.

   a. _____

   b. _____

   c. _____

2. Which of the following describe the functions of testosterone? (Select all that apply.)

   a. Maintain sexual libido
   b. Spermatogenesis
   c. Mammary gland functioning
   d. Body hair distribution
   e. Cause an erection

3. List the two stages of ejaculation.

   a. _____

   b. _____

4. Fertilization of an ovum usually occurs in which of the following structures?

   a. Fallopian tube
   b. Vagina
   c. Uterus
   d. Ovaries

5. The female body structure analogous to the male phallus is the:

   a. Vagina
   b. Cervix
   c. Clitoris
   d. Uterus

6. _____ glands secrete mucus, which may contribute to vaginal lubrication during sexual activity.

7. List the two physiological responses to effective sexual stimulation for both males and females.

   a. _____

   b. _____

8. In which phase of the sexual response cycle will the male testes increase over 50 percent in size?

   a. Excitement
   b. Plateau
   c. Orgasm
   d. Resolution

9. Which of the following are characteristics of the detumescence process within the male sexual response cycle? (Select all that apply.)

   a. Seminal fluid is expelled.
   b. Prostate gland constricts.
   c. Blood flow to the penis decreases.
   d. Pelvic floor muscles constrict.
   e. It concludes within 10 to 30 minutes after orgasm.

10. Which of the following classes of medications have been associated with sexual dysfunction? (Select all that apply.)

    a. Steroids
    b. Calcium channel blockers
    c. Beta blockers
    d. Diuretics
    e. Opiates

11. Which of the following helps facilitate a sexual health discussion between a client and a health care professional?

    a. Provide a pre-consultation questionnaire
    b. Ask if the client is having issues with sex
    c. Avoid discussing it unless the client brings it up
    d. Nothing

12. A female client who is experiencing intimate partner violence may demonstrate which of the following behaviors?

    a. Trust
    b. Questioning authority figures
    c. Cheerfulness
    d. Flat affect

13. Which of the following instructions should be given to a female client before having a Pap smear? (Select all that apply.)

    a. Avoid red meat 5 days before the test
    b. Schedule the test for 10 days after the last menstrual period
    c. No restrictions on the use of spermicidal foams
    d. Avoid douching for 2 days before the test
    e. No specific instructions

14. During the bimanual examination of the female pelvic organs, the uterus is _____ between the vagina and abdomen.

15. A 65-year-old male client's prostate-specific antigen (PSA) level is 3 nanograms. This finding indicates:

    a. Nothing
    b. Need for more testing
    c. Unusual elevation for the client's age
    d. Pending prostate cancer

16. The second cervical sample from a Pap smear is used to test for:

    a. Clamydia
    b. Gonorrhea
    c. Human papillomavirus (HPV)
    d. Syphilis

17. Which of the following mucous changes indicate ovulation has occurred in a female client? (Select all that apply.)

    a. Thin consistency
    b. Scant amount
    c. Thick consistency
    d. Sticky consistency
    e. Slippery consistency

18. Which of the following should the nurse instruct a client being treated for an STI?

    a. Nothing
    b. Avoid exercise
    c. Limit bathing
    d. Return for a re-test to check if the illness is cured

Female Reproductive Dysfunction: Nursing Management

1. Name the parts of the female athlete triad seen in reproductive dysfunction.

   a. _____
   b. _____
   c. _____

2. The period of 5 to 10 years before menses ends is called:

   a. Menarche
   b. Amenorrhea
   c. Perimenopause
   d. Menopause

3. Which of the following is a hallmark sign of premenstrual dysphoric disorder?

   a. Insomnia
   b. A symptom-free length of time every month
   c. Mood swings
   d. Food cravings

4. The most common endocrine disorder in women of childbearing age is _____ syndrome.

5. A 45-year-old female experiencing anovulatory bleeding should be evaluated for:

   a. Menopause
   b. Polyps
   c. Ovarian cysts
   d. Endometrial cancer

6. The only specific test to diagnose endometriosis is a(n):

   a. Laparoscopy
   b. Pelvic exam
   c. Ultrasound
   d. Follicle-stimulating hormone (FSH) blood level

7. Which of the following menstrual disorder hormone medications is used to treat endometriosis?

   a. Motrin
   b. Vaniqa
   c. Luvox
   d. Mirena

8. Which of the following are lifestyle modifications to relieve hot flashes? (Select all that apply.)

   a. Smoking cessation
   b. Avoid spicy foods
   c. Hypnotism
   d. Increase exercise
   e. Weight reduction
   f. Acupuncture

9. A client diagnosed with chronic candidal infections should be tested for: (Select all that apply.)

   a. Human papillomavirus (HPV)
   b. Diabetes
   c. Chronic obstructive pulmonary disorder (COPD)
   d. Human immunodeficiency virus (HIV)
   e. Asthma

10. What is HPV associated with?

    a. _____
    b. _____

11. Which of the following can be used to prevent candidal yeast infections?

    a. Prophylactic use of over the counter yeast infection medications
    b. Restrict dairy products
    c. Limit coffee
    d. Eat yogurt

12. After receiving a pelvic examination, a client is diagnosed with a prolapsed bladder. This finding is also called a(n):

    a. Urethrocele
    b. Cystocele
    c. Rectocele
    d. Enterocele

13. The most common solid pelvic tumors in women are uterine fibroids, or _____.

14. The diagnostic test that analyzes the interior fallopian tubes and uterus is a(n):

    a. Hysterosalpingogram
    b. Ultrasound
    c. Saline infusion sonogram
    d. Serum human chorionic gonadotropin (HCG) level

15. Performing Kegel exercises contracts the:

    a. Rectal muscles
    b. Pectoralis muscles
    c. Biceps muscles
    d. Pubococcygeus muscle

16. Which of the following structures are commonly removed during female circumcision? (Select all that apply.)

    a. Labia majora
    b. Cervix
    c. Labia minora
    d. Vagina
    e. Clitoris

17. List the four factors that influence the quality of life of people diagnosed with cancer.

    a. _____
    b. _____
    c. _____
    d. _____

18. The most commonly reported symptom of sexual dysfunction is:

    a. Decreased lubrication
    b. Hypoactive sexual desire
    c. Decreased ability to orgasm
    d. Pain with intercourse

CHAPTER 63

Breast Alterations: Nursing Management

1. The female breasts are supported by the pectoralis major muscle and by fibrous bands called _____ ligaments.

2. List the three major hormones that affect the breast.

    a. _____
    b. _____
    c. _____

3. A 17-year-old female complains of breast fullness and discomfort during her menstrual cycle. Which of the following should be done for this client?

    a. Schedule a mammogram
    b. Teach to restrict fluids during this time
    c. Suggest starting birth control pills
    d. Nothing. This is a common complaint.

4. A male client with enlarged breast tissue is experiencing _____.

5. Which of the following body postures facilitates the discovery of breast tissue dimpling?

    a. Press palms together
    b. Raise arms over the head
    c. Make a fist
    d. Lean forward

6. Which of the following is considered the last part of a breast examination?

    a. Client demonstrates breast self-examination
    b. Palpate the supraclavicular lymph nodes
    c. Assess for nipple discharge
    d. Palpate axillary lymph nodes

7. Which of the following are terms that describe breast pain? (Select all that apply.)

    a. Galactorrhea
    b. Mastodynia
    c. Mastalgia
    d. Mastitis
    e. Ectasia

8. List the three primary pathological conditions of the nipple.

   a. _____

   b. _____

   c. _____

9. Which of the following can cause galactorrhea? (Select all that apply.)

   a. Increased intake of vitamin D
   b. Blood pressure medications
   c. Low sodium intake
   d. Use of marijuana
   e. Hormone replacement therapy

10. A cancerous breast tumor appears as a(n) _____ area on a mammogram.

11. The surgical procedure to enlarge the breasts is called _____.

12. The most common complication of breast augmentation is:

   a. Capsular contracture
   b. Hematoma formation
   c. Infection
   d. Prosthesis leakage

13. From the following, choose those that enhance a women's potential for benign breast disease? (Select all that apply.)

   a. Alcohol consumption
   b. Obesity
   c. Breast feeding
   d. Age between 20 and 50 years
   e. Caffeine

14. Mammography is highly accurate and will detect what percentage of breast cancers in asymptomatic women?

   a. 90 percent
   b. 80 to 85 percent
   c. 70 to 75 percent
   d. 5 to 10 percent

15. The purpose of a breast ultrasound is to:

   a. Screen for breast cancer
   b. Determine mammary gland functioning
   c. Analyze normal breast tissue
   d. Characterize breast masses

16. The purpose of chemotherapy before surgery for breast cancer is to:

   a. Decrease tumor size
   b. Avoid surgery
   c. Kill cells that migrate to other body parts
   d. Reduce breast pain

17. Which of the following describes the simplest breast reconstruction that can occur at the time of a mastectomy?

   a. Transplant tissue to the mastectomy site
   b. Use of transverse rectus abdominis myocutaneous (TRAM) flap
   c. Use of free-flap reconstruction
   d. Use of saline-filled implants for reconstruction

CHAPTER 64

Male Reproductive Dysfunction: Nursing Management

1. A male client with a recurring infection of the prostate gland is experiencing what type of prostatitis?

   a. Acute
   b. Chronic
   c. Chronic bacterial
   d. Chronic pelvic pain syndrome

2. The medications of choice to treat bacterial prostatitis are: (Select all that apply.)

   a. Penicillin
   b. Doxycycline
   c. Amoxicillin
   d. Ampicillin
   e. Ciprofloxacin

3. Which of the following is used to differentiate benign prostatic hypertrophy (BPH) from prostate cancer? (Select all that apply.)

   a. Prostate-specific antigen (PSA) level
   b. Digital rectal exam
   c. Rectal ultrasound
   d. Intravenous pyelogram (IVP)
   e. Dihydrotestosterone (DHT) level

4. Which of the following surgical procedures for BPH improves urine flow and symptoms with few side effects?

   a. Transurethral resection of the prostate (TURP)
   b. Transurethral microwave procedure (TUMP)
   c. Transurethral needle ablation (TUNA)
   d. TURA

5. _____ cancer is the second most commonly diagnosed cancer in men.

6. The recommended treatment for early stage, potentially curable prostate cancer in a man with a life expectancy greater than 10 years is:

   a. Radiation therapy
   b. Brachytherapy
   c. Chemotherapy
   d. Radical prostatectomy

7. List the two types of testicular cancer.

   a. _____
   b. _____

8. Painless enlargement of a testis can indicate:

   a. Trauma
   b. Urinary tract infection
   c. Cyst
   d. Cancer

9. Testicular torsion is more common in men with a(n) _____ deformity in which the testicles swing inside the scrotum.

10. A male who has experienced mumps is prone to developing:

    a. Epididymitis
    b. Orchitis
    c. Prostatitis
    d. Hydrocele

11. The most important preoperative teaching for a client scheduled for a vasectomy is:

    a. Understanding the risk of infection
    b. Understanding the healing process
    c. Understanding the risk of bleeding
    d. Understanding sterilization is permanent

12. List the two treatments for scrotal varioceles.

    a. _____
    b. _____

13. Which of the following is an inflammation of the glans penis?

    a. Balanitis
    b. Posthitis
    c. Balanoposthitis
    d. Phimosis

14. A male client who has experienced multiple traumatic urinary catheterizations is prone to developing:

    a. Urethral stricture
    b. Urethritis
    c. Epispadias
    d. Hypospadias

15. A severely curved penis because of scar tissue in the corpora cavernosa is referred to as _____ disease.

16. Side effects of Viagra include: (Select all that apply.)

    a. Headache
    b. Flushing
    c. Palpitations
    d. Blue-tinged vision
    e. Dizziness

Special Considerations in Medical and Surgical Nursing

CHAPTER 65

Multisystem Failure

1. During the immune inflammatory response, the body cells switch from aerobic to anaerobic metabolism, which leads to what type of acid-base imbalance?

   a. Respiratory acidosis
   b. Respiratory alkalosis
   c. Metabolic acidosis
   d. Metabolic alkalosis

2. Which of the following is an uncontrolled acute inflammatory response that causes inflammation in multiple organs that are not the original site of injury?

   a. Systemic inflammatory response syndrome (SIRS)
   b. Acute respiratory distress syndrome (ARDS)
   c. Multiple organ dysfunction syndrome (MODS)
   d. Disseminated intravascular coagulation (DIC)

3. Which of the following should be included in the care of the client diagnosed with DIC? (Select all that apply.)

   a. Administer careful turning and repositioning
   b. Provide intramuscular injections for pain relief
   c. Encourage increasing activity
   d. Avoid intramuscular injections
   e. Provide stool softeners

4. List the three classifications of shock syndrome.

   a. _____
   b. _____
   c. _____
   d. _____

5. A client who is experiencing shock and whose body can no longer respond to therapy is in which stage of the shock syndrome?

   a. Initial
   b. Compensatory
   c. Multiple organ failure (MOF)
   d. Refractory

6. Into which type of shock syndrome should anaphylactic shock be categorized?

   a. Hypovolemic
   b. Distributive
   c. Obstructive
   d. Cardiogenic

7. Which of the following should be included when instructing a client prone to developing anaphylactic shock? (Select all that apply.)

    a. Ways to prevent the onset
    b. The best hospital to treat this type of shock
    c. How to obtain a medical alert bracelet
    d. Prepare and carry a list of allergies
    e. Ways to limit the intake of the offending allergen

8. A client who has sustained an acute myocardial infarction with 45 percent heart damage is prone to developing what type of shock?

    a. Anaphylactic
    b. Hypovolemic
    c. Cardiogenic
    d. Septic

9. List the three types of hypovolemic shock.

    a. _____
    b. _____
    c. _____

10. The use of red blood cells to treat hypovolemic shock can trigger:

    a. Anaphylactic shock
    b. Tachycardia
    c. Muscle cramping
    d. Nausea and vomiting

11. Which of the following are manifestations of neurogenic shock? (Select all that apply.)

    a. Hypertension
    b. Bradycardia
    c. Tachycardia
    d. Warm dry skin
    e. Hypotension

12. Which of the following can lead to the development of DIC?

    a. Cardiogenic shock
    b. Hypovolemic shock
    c. Septic shock
    d. Neurogenic shock

13. Which of the following can precipitate multisystem failure?

    a. Aspiration
    b. Kidney stone
    c. Pain
    d. Leg fracture

14. A client diagnosed with primary multiple-organ dysfunction and inflammation can develop:

    a. ARDS
    b. SIRS
    c. DIC
    d. Anaphylactic shock

15. Long-term treatment in an intensive care unit can lead to the development of:

    a. Pressure sores
    b. Contractures
    c. Stasis pneumonia
    d. Intensive care unit psychosis

Mass Casualty Care

1. The first step in the care of a client who arrives in an emergency department (ED) is to _____, or sort and assign the client a priority level for care.

2. Most EDs today use how many levels of care when triaging clients?

   a. I
   b. II
   c. III
   d. IV

3. Because of Emergency Medical Treatment and Labor Act (EMTALA) legislation, which of the following must occur for every person who arrives in an ED requesting treatment?

   a. Present proof of health insurance
   b. Claim next of kin
   c. Have a valid home phone number
   d. Conduct a medical screening examination

4. What does the mnemonic START mean?

   a. S = _____
   b. T = _____
   c. A = _____
   d. R = _____
   e. T = _____

5. Which of the following colors used to classify clients during a mass casualty incident means the client has minor injuries?

   a. Green
   b. Yellow
   c. Red
   d. Black

6. Incident command systems were originally created for which of the following industries?

   a. Law enforcement
   b. Car manufacturing
   c. Firefighting
   d. Chemical processing

7. List the four components of the hospital emergency incident command system.

   a. F = _____
   b. L = _____
   c. O = _____
   d. P = _____

8. Which of the following are components of expanded precautions (select all that apply)?

   a. Blood exposure
   b. Contact
   c. Droplet
   d. Non-intact skin
   e. Airborne

9. _____, or hazardous materials, have the potential to harm a person or the environment.

10. Hospital laboratory employees who have received vaccinations to prevent infection fall into which of the biological safety levels?

    a. Level I
    b. Level II
    c. Level III
    d. Level IV

11. The primary difference between chickenpox and smallpox is that the smallpox rash is more concentrated on the:

    a. Chest
    b. Abdomen
    c. Buttocks
    d. Face

12. List the three forms of the plague.

    a. _____
    b. _____
    c. _____

13. Which of the following is considered the greatest bioterrorism threat?

    a. Ebola
    b. Anthrax
    c. Severe acute respiratory syndrome (SARS)
    d. West Nile Virus (WNV)

14. The type of precaution needed when caring for a patient with West Nile Virus is:

    a. Contact
    b. Droplet
    c. Airborne
    d. Standard

15. The most common fatal injury seen in initial blast survivors is:

    a. Fracture
    b. Blast lung
    c. Closed head injury
    d. Traumatic amputation

16. A prolonged stress response that occurs after a traumatic event and can last for weeks or months is:

    a. Psychosis
    b. Neurosis
    c. Chronic fatigue syndrome
    d. Posttraumatic stress disorder

Answer Key

Chapter 1 Answers

1. B
2. Biotechnology
3. C
4. A
5. A, C, and D
6. Safety
7. B
8. A
9. C, A, B, and D
10. D
11. A, C, and D
12. Clinical practice, education, administration, and research
13. A, B, and C
14. A
15. A, C, and D
16. Terminal
17. C
18. D
19. A, B, and C
20. A

Chapter 2 Answers

1. Experience, trial and error, textbooks, research, procedure manuals
2. B
3. A
4. Science
5. A, E, B, C, and F
6. A and D
7. Evidence summary
8. A, B, C, and D
9. A, B, and D
10. B
11. Power, validity
12. B, C, and D
13. The Cochrane Collaboration, Agency for Healthcare Research and Quality
14. C
15. C

Chapter 3 Answers

1. B
2. Patient education
3. D
4. C
5. B
6. A
7. B
8. B and C
9. Assessment, diagnosis, goals, interventions, evaluation
10. B
11. Developmental stage
12. B
13. Motivational interviewing
14. C
15. A, C, and D
16. Health promotion
17. A
18. B and C
19. B
20. Evaluation of outcomes

Chapter 4 Answers

1. B, C, and D
2. Ethnic groups
3. Cultural shock
4. D
5. A
6. A, B, and C
7. Race
8. White
9. C
10. A
11. C
12. B
13. B
14. D
15. C
16. A
17. Objective, unbiased, and nonjudgmental
18. A, B, and D
19. C
20. A, B, and D

Chapter 5 Answers

1. B, C, and D
2. Ethics
3. Clinical ethics
4. A
5. C
6. B
7. C
8. American Nurses Association
9. Patient's Bill of Rights
10. D
11. A, C, and D
12. A and D
13. A
14. A, B, C, and D
15. B
16. A
17. Medical futility
18. B
19. A
20. A, B, C, and D

Chapter 6 Answers

1. B
2. C
3. Prevalence, incidence, trends
4. A
5. A, B, and C
6. C
7. A and B
8. A and B
9. A
10. D
11. D
12. C
13. Health
14. A, D, and E
15. A and D
16. B
17. A, B, and E

Chapter 7 Answers

1. Palliative care, curative treatment
2. C
3. C
4. B
5. A, B, and D
6. Willing caregiver
7. D
8. A, B, and C
9. A and C
10. Assisted suicide
11. A and D
12. A and B
13. B
14. A, B, C, and D
15. Euthanasia
16. D
17. C
18. A
19. B

Chapter 8 Answers

1. D
2. A
3. B, C, and D
4. D
5. B
6. A, D, and E
7. Physical assessment
8. D
9. Diaphragm
10. A, C, D, and E
11. B
12. A
13. D
14. Role
15. B
16. B, D, and E
17. Any five of the following: autonomy, benefi-cence, fidelity, justice, nonmaleficence, veracity
18. A
19. D

Chapter 9 Answers

1. B
2. C
3. B
4. Punnett square

5. C
6. Death, malformation, growth retardation, functional deficit
7. A, C, and D
8. D
9. A, C, D, and E
10. D
11. A
12. D

13. Forward genetics, positional genetics, candidate gene
14. C
15. D
16. Autonomy, beneficence, nonmaleficence, justice
17. Genetic Information Nondiscrimination Act (GINA)
18. B
19. B

Chapter 10 Answers

1. D
2. B, D, and F
3. Alarm reaction stage, stage of resistance, exhaustion stage
4. General Inhibition Syndrome
5. A
6. Any of the following may be listed: meditation, prayer, yoga, exercise, the "arts," acupuncture, acupressure, moxibustion, herbal medicine, ayurvedic medicine, homeopathic medicine, naturopathy, environmental medicines, culture-based medicines, diet, nutrition supplements, osteopathy, chiropractic medicine, massage, reflexology, therapeutic touch
7. C

8. D
9. B
10. Detachment, depersonalization, inability to cope
11. C
12. A
13. B
14. D
15. C
16. Roy = Adaptation model, Neuman = Systems model, Orem = Self-care theory
17. D
18. Cost containment module of managed care, evidence-based practice model, personal empowerment

Chapter 11 Answers

1. Neutrophils, monophils
2. B
3. Redness, swelling (edema), heat, pain
4. A
5. C
6. D
7. B, D, and E
8. Contact, droplet, airborne, common vehicle, vector borne
9. C, D, and E
10. B

11. A
12. A
13. C
14. B
15. Bleeding, hypovolemia, steroid drugs, decreased nutrition, and bio burden
16. B
17. Sensory perception, moisture, activity, mobility, nutrition, friction and shear
18. B

Chapter 12 Answers

1. Interstitial, intravascular, transcellular
2. B
3. A
4. C
5. Atrial natriuretic peptide
6. R = Renin, A = Angiotensin, A = Aldosterone, S = System

7. D
8. B
9. C
10. D
11. A
12. C
13. 3.5, 5.5

14. B

15. Trousseau's sign (carpopedal spasm), Chvostek's sign

16. B

17. B

18. D

19. Anion gap

20. PO_2 = 80–100 mm Hg, PCO_2 = 35–45 mm Hg, HCO_3 = 22–26 mEq/L, pH = 7.35–7.45, O_2 Sat = 97–100%

Chapter 13 Answers

1. Outer layer or tunica adventitia, middle layer or tunica media, inner layer or tunica intima
2. A
3. Dorsal metacarpal, cephalic, median, basilic
4. D
5. A, B, and E
6. B, C, and F
7. C
8. C and D
9. G = Give, D = Dose, H = Hand (on hand), V = Volume
10. 2.2
11. Dose, drug, patient, time, route
12. A
13. Continuous, intermittent, direct injection, patient-controlled analgesia
14. A, B, and E
15. B
16. A, D, and E
17. Thinner, dryer, subcutaneous
18. C, A, D, and B

Chapter 14 Answers

1. A, D, and E
2. B, C, and E
3. Naturopathy, homeopathy
4. China, Asian Indian, Greece, Native American, Egyptian
5. B
6. A, B, and E
7. C
8. A, C, and D
9. Qi, chi (vital energy), meridians
10. D
11. C
12. C
13. C
14. B
15. A
16. A, B, and D
17. Biofeedback
18. A
19. D

Chapter 15 Answers

1. Heredity, environment, lifestyle
2. A, C, and D
3. Initiation, promotion, progression, metastasis
4. A
5. CAUTION
6. C
7. Surgery, pharmacotherapy (or chemotherapy), radiation
8. Brachytherapy
9. D
10. B
11. Fatigue
12. D
13. Autologous, allogeneic, syngenic
14. A, B, and D
15. C
16. D
17. A
18. D
19. D

Chapter 16 Answers

1. Subjective, fifth
2. Specificity, pattern, gate control
3. A
4. B
5. D
6. D
7. A
8. Comprehensive assessment, consistent use of assessment tools, continuous reassessment, customized care plan, collaboration
9. A, C, and E
10. B, C, and D
11. B
12. D

13. B
14. Suffering, sleeplessness, sadness
15. D

16. A
17. D

Chapter 17 Answers

1. Pharmaceutic, pharmacokinetic, pharmacodynamic
2. A
3. C
4. Pharmacodynamics
5. D, A, C, F, B, and E
6. C
7. B
8. D
9. A

10. B
11. D
12. B and C,
13. C
14. D
15. D
16. A and D
17. C and D
18. A
19. B

Chapter 18 Answers

1. Cost, access, quality
2. A, D, and E
3. Availability, Accessibility, Accommodation, Affordability, Acceptability
4. Structure, process, outcome
5. Humanistic, financial, clinical
6. D
7. A
8. C and D
9. D
10. Adult daycare

11. A, C, and E
12. D
13. MDS (Minimum Data Set), OSCAR (Online Survey, Certification, and Reporting Systems)
14. B
15. Characteristics, competencies
16. B
17. S = Situation, B = Background, A = Assessment, R = Recommendation
18. C

Chapter 19 Answers

1. Generalized, specialized
2. B
3. A, D, and F
4. C
5. Reassurance, flexible visitation, information, comfort, support
6. B, D, and E
7. A and E
8. C
9. Blood clots, kinks, air bubbles, loose connections

10. D
11. 60
12. A, B, and D
13. D
14. Ventricular assist device
15. B
16. B
17. Sniffing
18. A
19. C
20. A, C, D, and F

Chapter 20 Answers

1. Diagnosis-related groups (DRGs), clinical pathways
2. Short-stay surgery
3. D
4. B, D, and E
5. A
6. D
7. Perioperative

8. C
9. C
10. A, D, and E
11. D
12. Opioids, amnesic muscle relaxants, anticholinergics, antacids or hydrogen ion antagonists
13. C, D, and F
14. Nonelective

15. B
16. A, C, and D

17. Autologous

Chapter 21 Answers

1. C
2. B and E
3. Intermediate
4. A
5. B, D, and E
6. Unrestricted, semirestricted, restricted
7. A
8. Sterilization, disinfection
9. A and C
10. D
11. Desiccate, fulgurate
12. C
13. Local, regional, spinal, epidural, general
14. B
15. B and E
16. Time out
17. A
18. A, B, D

Chapter 22 Answers

1. A, B, and D
2. C
3. D
4. B
5. A, D, and F
6. Bair hugger (Note to copyeditor: This is the correct spelling B-A-I-R.)
7. D
8. Penrose, Davol, Jackson Pratt (JP)
9. Aldrete system
10. C
11. A
12. Extremity warmth, color, pulses, capillary refill
13. B
14. D
15. C and D
16. C

Chapter 23 Answers

1. C
2. A and D
3. Bone marrow, erythropoiesis
4. B
5. Intrinsic, extrinsic
6. D
7. B, C, and E
8. A
9. Endocardium, myocardium, pericardium
10. A and D
11. C
12. C
13. D
14. Sternum, ribs, clavicles
15. Decrease
16. A
17. C, D, and E
18. D
19. A
20. C

Chapter 24 Answers

1. Daily fruit and vegetable consumption, alcohol intake, psychosocial index
2. D
3. C
4. B
5. Foam
6. A
7. Angina pectoris, acute coronary syndrome, sudden cardiac death
8. C
9. P = Precipitating event, Q = Quality, R = Radiation, S = Severity, T = Timing
10. Levine's
11. C and D
12. D
13. A
14. B
15. B and E
16. Transmyocardial laser
17. D
18. M = Morphine intravenous (IV) line, O = Oxygen, N = Nitroglycerin, A = Aspirin
19. Aspirin
20. A

Chapter 25 Answers

1. D
2. A
3. B and C
4. D
5. A, B, and F
6. Dilated, hypertrophic, arrhythmogenic (right ventricular), restrictive
7. Myectomy
8. A, D, and E
9. C
10. Endocarditis, myocarditis, pericarditis
11. Janeway
12. B, D, and E
13. Hypotension, elevated jugular pressure, muffled heart sounds
14. C
15. Transesophageal
16. A
17. B
18. C
19. B

Chapter 26 Answers

1. E, C, A, B, and D
2. AV
3. Automaticity, excitability, conductivity, contractility
4. C
5. Conduction system abnormalities, abnormal impulse generation
6. D
7. B and D
8. Wenckebach, Mobitz
9. C
10. Hypovolemia, hypoxia, hydrogen ion, hyper- or hypokalemia, hypothermia
11. D
12. R
13. A
14. Fixed, demand
15. B
16. A
17. C
18. A = Airway, B = Breathing, C = Circulation, D = Defibrillation
19. C
20. A, B, and F

Chapter 27 Answers

1. D
2. B
3. C, E, and F
4. B and C
5. Embolus
6. Pulseless, pain, pallor, paresthesia, paralysis, poikilothermia
7. B
8. D
9. A
10. Venous stasis, vessel wall injury, altered blood coagulation
11. Homan's
12. D
13. A
14. Bleeding
15. B
16. C
17. D
18. A and C

Chapter 28 Answers

1. Essential, idiopathic
2. C
3. A
4. A, D, and E
5. Pulse pressure
6. D
7. B
8. D
9. B
10. A, E, and F
11. End organ
12. D
13. DASH
14. D
15. Aerobic activity, flexibility exercises, strengthening exercises
16. B

Chapter 29 Answers

1. Reed-Sternberg
2. D
3. CHOP; cyclophosphamide, hydroxydaunomycin, Oncovin, and prednisone
4. Bleeding, hypoproliferative, hemolytic
5. B
6. Vaso-oclusive, aplastic, sequestration, hyperhemolytic
7. A, D, and F
8. C
9. Immune thrombocytopenia purpura (ITP), thrombotic thrombocytopenia purpura (TTP)
10. B
11. Erythromelalgia
12. C
13. B and E
14. A
15. Bone marrow
16. B
17. D
18. Philadelphia
19. C
20. A

Chapter 30 Answers

1. A and E
2. Dead space
3. B
4. D
5. $PaCO_2$
6. C
7. B
8. Buffer system, pulmonary system, renal system
9. D
10. pH = 7.35–7.45; PaO_2 = 80–100 mmHg; $PaCO_2$ = 35–45 mm Hg; HCO_3 = 22–26 mm Hg
11. A
12. C
13. Residual volume
14. A
15. V = Ventilation, O = Obstruction, P = Protection, S = Secretions
16. B and C
17. D
18. C
19. Pulmonary emboli
20. B

Chapter 31 Answers

1. Allergic shiner, allergic crease, allergic salute
2. A and E
3. B
4. C
5. Rhinitis medicamentosa
6. B, C, and E
7. D
8. A
9. C
10. Quinsy, hot
11. A
12. Obstructive, central, mixed
13. B
14. Dryness
15. A and D
16. Heimlich
17. C
18. A
19. D
20. D

Chapter 32 Answers

1. Cough, dyspnea, hemoptysis
2. D
3. A, C, D, and F
4. B
5. Blastomycosis, histoplasmosis, aspergillus
6. B, C, and E
7. Cylindrical, varicose, cystic
8. D
9. T = Tumor, N = Node, M = Metastasis
10. B
11. Spontaneous, traumatic, iatrogenic, tension
12. C
13. B
14. B and E
15. Primary, secondary
16. A and E
17. D
18. A and D

Chapter 33 Answers

1. C
2. Puffers, bloaters
3. A, D, and E
4. A
5. B
6. C
7. A, B, and D
8. D
9. A
10. B

11. A
12. B and D
13. Green = Go, Yellow = Caution, Red = Stop
14. B
15. B, C, and F
16. Barotrauma
17. C
18. Lung transplant
19. A

Chapter 34 Answers

1. Neurons, neuroglial
2. D
3. B, C, and E
4. D
5. B
6. Brain, spinal cord
7. Cervical = 7, Thoracic = 12, Lumbar = 5, Sacral = 5 (fused 1), Coccygeal = 4 (fused 1)
8. D
9. A
10. B, C, and E

11. Oculomotor (CN III), vagus (CN X)
12. A, B, and D
13. Eye opening, verbal response, best motor response
14. B
15. C
16. A
17. C
18. Lumbar puncture
19. A
20. D

Chapter 35 Answers

1. Ischemic, hemorrhagic
2. B, D, and E
3. A
4. D
5. A and D
6. B
7. Motor vehicle
8. C
9. Mild, moderate, severe
10. A

11. A, D, and E
12. B
13. Intracranial
14. D
15. Glioma
16. A and E
17. Surgery, radiation, chemotherapy
18. A
19. C

Chapter 36 Answers

1. B
2. C
3. Brown-Séquard
4. A, B, and E
5. D
6. Halo
7. B
8. A and D
9. Autonomic dysreflexia
10. A

11. C
12. D
13. Extramedullary
14. D
15. Ophthalmic, maxillary, mandibular
16. B
17. Bell's palsy
18. D
19. D

Chapter 37 Answers

1. A
2. Tension, migraine, cluster
3. D
4. A, D, and F
5. B
6. B and C
7. Prodromal, aural, ictal, postictal
8. D
9. B
10. B and F
11. C
12. A
13. T = Tremors, R = Rigidity, A = Akinesia, P = Postural disturbance
14. B
15. C
16. A
17. B
18. Locked-in
19. D

Chapter 38 Answers

1. B
2. B, C, and E
3. A
4. Corneal
5. Superior nasal, inferior nasal, superior temporal, inferior temporal
6. D
7. C
8. Direct, consensual
9. A and E
10. Otorrhea
11. D
12. B and C
13. D
14. C
15. B, D, and F

Chapter 39 Answers

1. Strabismus, nystagmus, ocular muscle paralysis
2. A
3. Nystagmus
4. B, D, and F
5. C
6. Disease, personal behavior, medical treatment, environment
7. A and B
8. C
9. Closed-angle
10. A
11. B
12. Cryopexy
13. C
14. Abrasions, ulcerations, keratoconus
15. D
16. A
17. C and E
18. B
19. D
20. C

Chapter 40 Answers

1. B, C, and E
2. Inner
3. D
4. Conductive, sensorineural, mixed
5. A, D, and E
6. A
7. B
8. Presbycusis
9. C
10. D
11. B and D
12. Schwartz
13. D
14. B
15. Cochlear
16. B
17. B and E
18. Analog, digital

Chapter 41 Answers

1. Mechanical, chemical, microbial
2. D
3. A
4. Cell-mediated

5. B and E
6. Neutralization, opsonization, activation of inflammation, activation of complement
7. Cytokines
8. C
9. D
10. B

11. D
12. C, D, and E
13. B, C, and F
14. A
15. A and D
16. B and E
17. Anergy

Chapter 42 Answers

1. Vaginal delivery, breastfeeding
2. A, B, and E
3. C
4. B
5. D
6. B, D, and F
7. Highly active antiretroviral therapy
8. B
9. Initiation, immune response, inflammatory, destruction

10. A
11. B and C
12. C, E, and F
13. D
14. B
15. B, C, and D
16. C = Calcinosis, R = Raynaud's syndrome, E = Esophageal movement, S = Sclerodactyly, T = Telangiectasia

Chapter 43 Answers

1. Defense, homeostasis, surveillance
2. B
3. B
4. A, C, and E
5. Atopy
6. A, B, and C
7. D
8. C

9. Speed
10. A
11. Ragweed
12. C
13. A, D, and E
14. D
15. B

Chapter 44 Answers

1. Epidermis, dermis
2. B, C, and D
3. Subcutaneous
4. A
5. A, B, and D
6. Sebum
7. D
8. C
9. Lentigines

10. Inflammation, proliferation, maturation
11. A
12. Pseudomonas
13. B
14. A and E
15. D
16. Mohs'
17. D

Chapter 45 Answers

1. Mechanical, enzymatic, autolytic, sharp
2. A
3. C
4. Moisture-retentive
5. B
6. Irritant, allergic
7. D
8. A and D
9. Basal cell, squamous cell

10. A, B, and D
11. D
12. Cellulitis
13. A
14. B
15. C
16. C
17. D

Chapter 46 Answers

1. Heat, chemicals, electricity, radiation
2. C
3. Coagulation, stasis, hyperemia
4. A
5. Stop
6. D
7. B
8. B, C, and F
9. A
10. A
11. Escharotomy
12. B, D, and E
13. D
14. C
15. Urine output
16. B
17. Any four of the following: withdrawal, denial, regression, anger or hostility, depression, anxiety
18. D
19. Therapeutic positioning
20. B and C

Chapter 47 Answers

1. B and D
2. Three
3. Duodenum, jejunum, ileum
4. A and E
5. C
6. D
7. B, C, and E
8. B, D, C, and A
9. Cullen's
10. A and D
11. A
12. C
13. D
14. B, D, and E
15. B

Chapter 48 Answers

1. Tobacco use, improper diet, physical inactivity
2. C
3. D
4. A
5. Cytochrome P-450s
6. B, C, and D
7. C
8. B and C
9. A
10. Marasmus
11. C
12. D
13. A
14. B
15. Dumping syndrome
16. D

Chapter 49 Answers

1. Borborygmi
2. C
3. A and D
4. Videofluoroscopy
5. D
6. Compensatory techniques, indirect therapy, direct therapy
7. A
8. C and E
9. Sliding, paraesophageal
10. A, C, and D
11. B
12. Three
13. D
14. B
15. C and D

Chapter 50 Answers

1. D
2. A
3. Digestion, absorption
4. B, C, and E
5. Appendicitis and small bowel obstruction
6. Inflammation, obstruction, vascular
7. B
8. A, B, and D
9. Tenesmus
10. B and C
11. A
12. C

13. D
14. B
15. C, D, and F

16. Crohn's disease, ulcerative colitis
17. A

Chapter 51 Answers

1. Lobule
2. D
3. Preicteric, icteric, posticteric
4. B
5. A
6. C, D, and F
7. Ascites
8. B and E

9. D
10. Hepatomegaly
11. A
12. A, D, and E
13. Orthotopic, auxiliary
14. B
15. D
16. A and E

Chapter 52 Answers

1. Kidneys, ureters, bladder, urethra
2. Retroperitoneal
3. D
4. B
5. A and D
6. Nephron
7. B and C
8. A

9. B, C, and E
10. One
11. C
12. A
13. Catheterization, bladder scan
14. D
15. Dysuria

Chapter 53 Answers

1. Upper, lower
2. A, D, and E
3. B and C
4. D
5. Nocturia
6. Ulcerative, nonulcerative
7. D
8. A
9. A, C, and D
10. Proteinuria, hypoalbuminemia, hypercholesterolemia

11. B
12. C
13. Urolithiasis, nephrolithiasis
14. B, D, and E
15. A
16. D
17. Renal artery stenosis, renal vein thrombosis, nephrosclerosis
18. A
19. B
20. Stress, urge, overflow, functional

Chapter 54 Answers

1. Pyelonephritis
2. A
3. B and D
4. D
5. A
6. X-linked dominant, autosomal recessive, autosomal dominant
7. C
8. B

9. A
10. Prerenal, intrarenal, postrenal
11. A and D
12. B and E
13. Five
14. C
15. Dialysis, renal transplant, do nothing
16. D
17. C

Chapter 55 Answers

1. Hormones
2. C
3. A, D, and E
4. B
5. C
6. C
7. Hypothalamus
8. A
9. D and E
10. Triiodothyronine
11. A
12. Alpha, beta, delta, F
13. B
14. D
15. Exophthalmos

Chapter 56 Answers

1. A
2. Acromegaly
3. B
4. A
5. B, C, and E
6. C
7. B and C
8. Addison's
9. D
10. B
11. Pheochromocytoma
12. B
13. Any five of the following: invasive, infarction, infiltrative, injury, iatrogenic, infections, idiopathic, isolated, immunological
14. A and E
15. C
16. A, C, and D
17. B
18. C
19. B, C, and E
20. Calcium

Chapter 57 Answers

1. Type 1, type 2, gestational
2. A
3. A, D, and E
4. Polydipsia, polyphagia, polyuria
5. C
6. B
7. D
8. B, D, A, and C
9. A
10. Hypoglycemia
11. Lipodystrophy
12. A
13. C
14. Fruity
15. C
16. Hypoglycemia unawareness
17. A, D, and E
18. Autonomic, sensorimotor (peripheral)
19. C

Chapter 58 Answers

1. Flat, short (cuboidal), long, irregular
2. B
3. D
4. A
5. C
6. Osteopenia
7. B
8. Synarthrosis, amphiarthrosis, diarthrosis
9. A, C, and E
10. B and D
11. Displaced fracture
12. D
13. Stance (weight bearing), swing (non–weight bearing)
14. C
15. A
16. Dual-energy X-ray absorptiometry

Chapter 59 Answers

1. Osteoarthritis
2. A and D
3. B
4. C and E
5. C

6. NSAIDs, gout medications, corticosteroids, analgesics
7. Erythema migrans
8. A and D
9. B
10. D
11. Elevated muscle enzymes, abnormal electromyogram, positive results from a muscle biopsy

12. C
13. A
14. A and E
15. B, C, and D
16. Osteomyelitis, three
17. A
18. B
19. Bending forward

Chapter 60 Answers

1. R = Rest, I = Ice, C = Compression, E = Elevation
2. B, C, and E
3. A and E
4. A
5. Tinel's sign, Phalen's maneuver
6. B and C
7. A
8. B
9. B and E
10. Achilles

11. C
12. D
13. D
14. B
15. Complete, incomplete
16. C
17. A and B
18. A
19. A, C, and D
20. B

Chapter 61 Answers

1. Produce sperm, transport sperm to the female reproductive tract, secrete testosterone
2. A, B, and D
3. Emission, expulsion
4. A
5. C
6. Bartholin's
7. Vasocongestion, myotonia
8. B
9. C and D

10. A, D, and E
11. A
12. D
13. B and D
14. Trapped
15. A
16. C
17. A and E
18. D

Chapter 62 Answers

1. Menstrual disorder, eating disorder, decreased bone mineral density
2. C
3. B
4. Polycystic ovary
5. D
6. A
7. D
8. A, D, and E
9. B and D

10. Genital warts, cervical cancer
11. D
12. B
13. Leiomyomata
14. A
15. D
16. C and E
17. Physical, social, psychological, spiritual
18. B

Chapter 63 Answers

1. Cooper's
2. Estrogen, progesterone, prolactin
3. D
4. Gynecomastia

5. B
6. A
7. B and C
8. Bleeding, discharge, fissures

9. B, D, and E
10. White
11. Breast augmentation
12. A
13. D and E

14. B
15. D
16. A
17. D

Chapter 64 Answers

1. C
2. B and E
3. A and C
4. C
5. Prostate
6. D
7. Germinal, nongerminal
8. D

9. Bell clapper
10. B
11. D
12. Varicocelectomy, embolization
13. A
14. B
15. Peyronie's
16. A, B, and D

Chapter 65 Answers

1. C
2. A
3. A, D, and E
4. Hypovolemic, cardiogenic, distributive
5. D
6. B
7. A, C, and D
8. C

9. Absolute, relative, third spacing
10. A
11. B, D, and E
12. C
13. A
14. B
15. D

Chapter 66 Answers

1. Triage
2. C
3. D
4. S = Simple, T = Triage, A = And, R = Rapid, T = Treatment
5. A
6. C
7. F = Finance, L = Logistics, O = Operations, P = Planning

8. B, C, and E
9. HazMats
10. B
11. D
12. Bubonic, septicemic, pneumonic
13. B
14. D
15. B
16. D